Government Responses to the COVID-19 Pandemic

Olga Shvetsova
Editor

Government Responses to the COVID-19 Pandemic

Between a Rock and a Hard Place

palgrave
macmillan

Editor
Olga Shvetsova
Binghamton University
NY, USA

ISBN 978-3-031-30843-7   ISBN 978-3-031-30844-4 (eBook)
https://doi.org/10.1007/978-3-031-30844-4

© The Editor(s) (if applicable) and The Author(s), under exclusive licence to Springer Nature Switzerland AG 2023
This work is subject to copyright. All rights are solely and exclusively licensed by the Publisher, whether the whole or part of the material is concerned, specifically the rights of translation, reprinting, reuse of illustrations, recitation, broadcasting, reproduction on microfilms or in any other physical way, and transmission or information storage and retrieval, electronic adaptation, computer software, or by similar or dissimilar methodology now known or hereafter developed.
The use of general descriptive names, registered names, trademarks, service marks, etc. in this publication does not imply, even in the absence of a specific statement, that such names are exempt from the relevant protective laws and regulations and therefore free for general use.
The publisher, the authors, and the editors are safe to assume that the advice and information in this book are believed to be true and accurate at the date of publication. Neither the publisher nor the authors or the editors give a warranty, expressed or implied, with respect to the material contained herein or for any errors or omissions that may have been made. The publisher remains neutral with regard to jurisdictional claims in published maps and institutional affiliations.

Cover illustration: © Alex Linch shutterstock.com

This Palgrave Macmillan imprint is published by the registered company Springer Nature Switzerland AG.
The registered company address is: Gewerbestrasse 11, 6330 Cham, Switzerland

Paper in this product is recyclable.

Abstract

As the world enters the era of increased frequency of global health and natural disasters under the looming threat of a changing climate, how we govern ourselves matters for the ways in which we will live through these difficult times. Authors in this volume share their observations backed with mixed methods of analysis on the many ways in which government organization and political realities affect crisis response and crisis management. First and foremost, the impact of constitutions, political regimes, and political institutions on crisis responsiveness is identifiable, in both small n and large N analysis, despite the many idiosyncrasies of individual country cases. Second, institutional history matters—provisions, put in place either recently, following a crisis, or long ago and almost forgotten through nonuse, come into play and either impede or empower decision makers, depending on how congruent they are with the de facto decision framework. Third, the economy imposes constraints on managing crises. The per-capita income, the structure of the economy, the condition of the labor force, and accumulated social capital all constitute prerequisites for formulating a more effective response. Fourth, political concerns of the day can make a huge difference: crisis response might be delayed because of political expediency, or it might be hijacked and repurposed to solidify the position of political incumbents. For a country, to enter a crisis without having its proverbial house in order, poses considerable dangers. Fifth, who does what in government—or the allocation of responsibilities—has revealed itself to be a living, breathing process. Such a process often undergoes rapid adjustments in times of crisis. Finally, and perhaps most importantly, all these influences affect the way governments respond to crises by shaping the incentives of the key decision makers to act and to take the risks associated with leadership during periods of hardship. The resolve of politicians to safeguard public health cannot be taken for granted, and their strategies should be scrutinized at least as much through a political lens as from the standpoint of public health benefits.

Keywords: COVID-19; Governments; Executives; Policies; Public health; Nonmedical interventions; Federalism; Elections; Institutions; Constitutions; Blame avoidance; Credit claiming; Global

Competing Interests
None of the authors has a conflict of interest to declare.

CONTENTS

1 **What the World has Learned About Their Governments During the COVID-19 Pandemic**   1
Olga Shvetsova

2 **The Institutional Underpinnings of Policymaking in the Face of the COVID-19 Pandemic in Europe**   17
William B. Heller, Ezgi Muftuoglu, and Dina Rosenberg

3 **An Analysis of Government Responses to COVID-19 in Latin America's Three Federations**   49
Julie VanDusky-Allen

4 **COVID-19 Response in India, Pakistan, and Bangladesh: Shared History, Different Processes**   75
Abdul Basit Adeel and Andrei Zhirnov

5 **Center-Regional Political Risk Sharing in the COVID-19 Public Health Crisis: Nigeria and South Africa**   107
Onsel Gurel Bayrali

6 **Pick Your Poison: Political Expediencies, Economic Necessities, and COVID-19 Response in Malaysia and Indonesia**   127
TianYi Zhao

vii

viii CONTENTS

7 Populist Responses to COVID-19: Turkey and Israel as Cases of Proscience Populism and the United States and Brazil as Examples of Science-Skeptic Populism   147
Mert Can Bayar and Didem Seyis

8 The Visegrad Populist Leaders' Responses to COVID-19 Pandemic   177
Hyoungrohk Chu

9 Common Law Systems and COVID-19 Policy Response: Protective Public Health Policy in the United States, Canada, New Zealand, and Australia   197
Michael Catalano and Aaron Chan

10 Commonalities and Differences in Governments' COVID-19 Public Health Responses Around the World   223
Olga Shvetsova and Andrei Zhirnov

Appendix A: Protective Policy Index (PPI) Policy Categories and Assigned Weights (Tables A.1 and A.2)   243

Appendix B: Power Sharing and Stringency of Nonmedical Interventions (Nmis) (Figs. B.1, B.2, B.3, and B.4)   245

Index   249

Notes on Contributors

Abdul Basit Adeel is a political sociologist enrolled in the Sociology and Social Data Analytics program at The Pennsylvania State University. His collaborative work has appeared in *Nature Scientific Data, Canadian Public Policy, Frontiers in Political Science,* and the *Journal of Political Institutions and Political Economy.*

Mert Can Bayar is a postdoctoral scholar at the Center for an Informed Public at the University of Washington. With a research focus on public opinion, he explores conspiracy theories and evolving attitudes pertinent to democracy and autocracy. His work straddles the interdisciplinary space between political psychology and comparative political behavior.

Onsel Gurel Bayrali is a Ph.D. candidate at the State University of New York at Binghamton. His work in comparative public policy and political economy focuses on the strategic behavior of political incumbents as they minimize their electoral risks via intergovernmental task sharing during crisis management.

Michael Catalano is a Ph.D. candidate in political science at the State University of New York at Binghamton. His research and teaching interests explore the motivations of majoritarian institutions (i.e., legislatures, executives, political parties, and nomination and selection systems) to constrain or empower courts as well as the implications of those actions for judicial behavior. He has published in such outlets as *Political Research Quarterly, Justice System Journal,* and *Journal of Political Institutions and Political Economy.*

x   NOTES ON CONTRIBUTORS

Aaron Chan is the Ronald O. Perelman Emergency Medicine Division of Health Equity, Diversity, and Inclusion Program Coordinator. Aaron's efforts have led to the continuous development of NYU's Emergency Medicine health equity initiatives. His primary focus has been to improve access to health care, public health, and public policy for New York City's neediest patients. With a strong background in program development, community outreach, and collaborative leadership, he is dedicated to promoting a diverse and compassionate healthcare landscape for all.

Hyoungrohk Chu is a Ph.D. candidate in the Department of Political Science at the State University of New York at Binghamton. With an interest in European party politics, he focuses on election and voting behavior, democratic representation and backsliding, and the role of political ideologies. His current research revolves around how political ideologies, such as populism, Euroscepticism, and illiberalism, influence individual-level voting behavior. His works have been published in *Scientific Data* (*Nature*) and *Democratic Society and Policy Studies* (Korean).

William B. Heller is Associate Professor in the Department of Political Science at the State University of New York at Binghamton. Professor Heller uses formal modeling and game-theoretic analysis to study the effects of political institutions on collective decision-making and behavior, focusing primarily on political parties. He has published in a number of journals, including the *American Journal of Political Science, Comparative Political Studies, Legislative Studies Quarterly,* and the *European Journal of Political Research.*

Ezgi Muftuoglu is a Ph.D. candidate at Binghamton University specializing in the study of comparative political parties and institutions. She has published on parties, institutions, and public health policy.

Dina Rosenberg is a research associate at the Center on Democratic Performance at the State University of New York at Binghamton. Prior to this, she held a tenured position as an Assistant Professor of Political Science at the School of Politics and Governance at the Higher School of Economics in Moscow. Her main research areas are comparative political economy, healthcare politics, innovations, and post-communist states. Her work has appeared in *Democratization, Post-Soviet Affairs, Social Science Research, Review of Policy Research, Economic Systems,* and other journals.

NOTES ON CONTRIBUTORS   xi

Didem Seyis is a Ph.D. candidate in Political Science at State University of New York at Binghamton and a research assistant at Johns Hopkins University. Her research focuses on democratic backsliding, populism, voting behavior, and identity politics. She has published in such peer-reviewed journals as *Nature, Political Studies, Electoral Studies, Journal of Political Institutions and Political Economy, Frontiers in Political Science,* and *Turkish Studies.*

Olga Shvetsova is Professor of Political Science and Economics at the State University of New York at Binghamton. She studies political institutions and political economy and is an author of a number of books and articles on constitutional political economy, strategic analysis, parties, federalism, and the politics of health.

Julie VanDusky-Allen is Assistant Professor of Political Science in the School of Public Service at Boise State University in Boise, Idaho. Her research centers on institutions, political parties, and government responses to COVID-19. Her work has appeared in *Political Research Quarterly, Comparative Political Studies,* and *Canadian Public Policy,* among others.

TianYi Zhao is a Ph.D. candidate at the State University of New York at Binghamton and focuses in his research on comparative politics and international relations. His primary areas of interest include multilevel governance, autocracies, collective identity formation, state-society relations, and the philosophy of social science, with a specialized area focus on East Asia and Southeast Asia.

Andrei Zhirnov is Lecturer in Quantitative Political Science at the University of Exeter. Dr. Zhirnov is a comparativist using statistical modeling to study political institutions and behavior. His work has appeared in such outlets as the *American Journal of Political Science, Journal of Political Institutions and Political Economy, Electoral Studies, Political Analysis,* and *Comparative Politics.*

LIST OF FIGURES

Fig. 1.1	Global variation in policy responsiveness during pandemic onset stage by level of government and by federal versus unitary type of government, on April 30, 2020. (Source: Shvetsova et al. (2022c)) 10
Fig. 2.1	Daily new COVID-19 cases per million residents in Denmark, Finland, Italy, and Spain. (Source: Mathieu E et al. (2020) Coronavirus Pandemic (COVID-19). Our World in Data, Oxford. https://ourworldindata.org/coronavirus) 26
Fig. 2.2	Covid impact and early responses in Denmark, Finland, Italy, and Spain: stringency and timing. (Source for stringency: Shvetsova et al. 2022; source for Deaths/million and Cases/million: Mathieu E et al. (2020) Coronavirus Pandemic (COVID-19). Our World in Data, Oxford. https://ourworldindata.org/coronavirus) 28
Fig. 3.1	PPI in Argentina, Mexico, and Brazil, January to December 2020. (Source: Shvetsova et al. 2022) 51
Fig. 4.1	Dynamics of infection outbreak and policy response in India, Pakistan, and Bangladesh, 2020. (Source: Shvetsova et al. 2022) 87
Fig. 4.2	Phases of COVID-19 pandemic response in 2020 88
Fig. 4.3	Timing of national lockdowns in India, Pakistan, and Bangladesh. (Source: Shvetsova et al. 2022) 93
Fig. 4.4	Institutional trajectories of epidemic response systems in India, Pakistan, and Bangladesh 100
Fig. 5.1	Public health policy stringencies (left) and national governments' policy involvement (right) in Nigeria and South Africa. (Source: Shvetsova et al. 2022) 109

xiv   LIST OF FIGURES

Fig. 7.1   Daily national (federal) PPI in Brazil, Israel, Turkey, and USA, year 2020. (Here we use national/federal PPI rather than total since our argument relies on national/federal level of responses to the pandemic. For a comparison and discussion on the national versus total PPI, please refer to the online appendix.) (Source: Shvetsova et al. 2022)   156

Fig. 7.2   Comparison of stringency of policies on individual location restrictions in Brazil, Israel, Turkey, and the USA, as measured by national PPI (*top*) and total PPI (*bottom*). (Source: Shvetsova et al. 2022)   164

Fig. 7.3   Comparison of stringency of restrictions in places of congregation in Brazil, Israel, Turkey, and the USA, as measured by national PPI (*top*) and total PPI (*bottom*). (Source: Shvetsova et al. 2022)   165

Fig. 8.1   Level of government protective policies (2020). (Source: Oxford Coronavirus Government Response Tracker (OxCGRT) (2022). Note: The Stringency Index (SI), the mean score of the following pandemic-relevant policy areas, is computed on a daily basis and thus points to how strict a set of COVID-19 nonpharmaceutical policies are: school closures, workplace closures, cancellation of public events, restriction on public gatherings, closures of public transport, stay-at-home requirements, public information campaigns, restrictions on internal movement, and international travel controls. A high SI score does not always suggest that a certain government's pandemic responses are excellent, but we can estimate whether their policy stringency is timely and sufficient especially in the absence of vaccination in 2020)   184

Fig. 10.1   Daily (Average Total) Protective Policy Index in Federal versus Unitary Countries, February–August 2020. (Source: Shvetsova et al. (2022), Freedom House (2020); author coding of federations.)   226

Fig. 10.2   NMI policy efforts of national and subnational governments on four dates in 2020. (Source: Shvetsova et al. (2022), Freedom House (2020); author coding of federations.)   227

Fig. 10.3   Relative policy contribution to overall NMI stringency by national and subnational governments on four dates in 2020. (Source: Shvetsova et al. (2022), Freedom House (2020); author coding of federations.)   228

Fig. 10.4   Protective policy stringency (average total PPI) and decentralization and federalism, April and June 2020. (Source: Shvetsova et al. (2022), Freedom House (2020),

	Shair-Rosenfield et al. (2020), Hooghe et al. (2016); author coding of federations.)	231
Fig. 10.5	Daily (average total) PPI in free, partly free, and nonfree countries, February–August 2020. (Source: Shvetsova et al. (2022), Freedom House (2020).)	232
Fig. 10.6	Daily (average total) PPI by country income group, February–August 2020. (Source: Shvetsova et al. (2022); the country income group is computed using gross national income (GNI) per capita, PPP (The World Bank, World Development Indicators 2020).)	235
Fig. 10.7	Daily (average total) PPI in countries with different healthcare financing models, February–August 2020. (Sources: Shvetsova et al. (2022), Freedom House (2020); author coding of healthcare models.)	236
Fig. 10.8	Government per-capita healthcare spending in 2019 and the protective policy stringency (average total) in April and June 2020. (Sources: Shvetsova et al. (2022), World Health Organization (2020a).)	237
Fig. 10.9	Doctors and nurses per 10,000 people in 2019 and the protective policy stringency (average total) in April and June 2020. (Sources: Shvetsova et al. (2022), World Health Organization (2020b).)	238
Fig. 10.10	Daily (average total) PPI in countries with and without a constitutionally specified right to health, February–August 2020. (Sources: Shvetsova et al. (2022), Freedom House (2020); author coding of constitutional responsibility for health.)	239
Fig. B.1	Daily (average total) Protective Policy Index in parliamentary (dotted) and presidential democracies, February–August 2020. (Source: Shvetsova et al. 2022)	245
Fig. B.2	NMI stringency and power sharing in national executive. (Sources: Shvetsova et al. 2022; Döring, Huber, and Manow 2022)	246
Fig. B.3	NMI stringency and multiparty systems in national legislatures, parliamentary democracies only. (Sources: Shvetsova et al. 2022; Döring et al. 2022)	246
Fig. B.4	Correspondence between annual mortality from airborne infections (per 100,000) and NMI stringency, in countries with rising and declining mortality rates, in April and June 2020. (Sources: Shvetsova et al. 2022; WHO Mortality Database 2022)	247

LIST OF TABLES

Table 2.1	Physicians, nurses, and hospital beds per 100,000 inhabitants in Denmark, Finland, Italy, and Spain	25
Table 2.2	Healthcare spending in Denmark, Finland, Italy, and Spain, 2019	25
Table 2.3	Parliamentary and cabinet parties in Denmark, Finland, Italy, and Spain	27
Table 3.1	Development Indicators Immediately Prior to the Pandemic in Argentina, Brazil, and Mexico	54
Table 3.2	Political Indicators Immediately Prior to the Pandemic in Argentina, Brazil, and Mexico	55
Table 3.3	Brazilian State-Level COVID-19 Policies (Robust Standard Errors in Parentheses)	61
Table 3.4	Mexican State-Level COVID-19 Policies (Robust Standard Errors in Parentheses)	68
Table 4.1	Feasible types of action in response to an infectious disease outbreak	78
Table 4.2	Differences in health crisis response structures in India, Pakistan, and Bangladesh	86
Table 5.1	Snapshot of COVID-19 pandemic in some African countries	112
Table 7.1	Comparison of Regime Type, Government Strength, and GDP per capita in Brazil, Israel, Turkey, and USA	157
Table 7.2	Comparison of National and Total PPI, Mortality, and Healthcare Institutions in Brazil, Israel, Turkey, and USA	159
Table 8.1	A theoretical framework for V4's pandemic handling in 2020	180
Table 8.2	Economic/health/political indicators in the Visegrad Group	186
Table 9.1	Political party systems and ideology in Settler British Commonwealth countries	204

xvii

xviii   LIST OF TABLES

Table 9.2	Ideological identification of Supreme Court of United States in 2020	206
Table 9.3	Ideological identification of Supreme Court of Canada in 2020	206
Table 9.4	Ideological identification of Supreme Court of New Zealand in 2020	207
Table 9.5	Ideology identification of the High Court of Australia in 2020	208
Table 9.6	Counts of COVID-19 policy response cases decided on the merits in 2020	214
Table A.1	Policy categories and their weights in PPI construction, method 1	243
Table A.2	Policy categories and their weights in Protective Policy Index construction, method 2	244

CHAPTER 1

What the World has Learned About Their Governments During the COVID-19 Pandemic

Olga Shvetsova

1.1 Introduction

In early 2020, initial reports appeared in the media about a new deadly disease that was ravaging the city of Wuhan in Hubei Province of China. By the end of January, Chinese authorities had instituted lockdowns and quarantines and started sharing information about the disease, SARS-CoV-2, which came to be known as COVID-19. The virus proved very transmissible and spread globally fairly quickly (Hsiang et al. 2020), showing up in the Americas, Europe, and the Middle East as early as February. It was established eventually, but not immediately, that it spread by airborne transmission, and reliable diagnostic materials were initially very scarce. Pulmonary and gastrointestinal symptoms were often followed by severe complications and death, and existing treatments were of little help. Because the proper tests for identifying asymptomatic cases did not yet

O. Shvetsova (✉)
Department of Political Science, Binghamton University, Binghamton, NY, USA
e-mail: shvetso@binghamton.edu

© The Author(s), under exclusive license to Springer Nature
Switzerland AG 2023
O. Shvetsova (ed.), *Government Responses to the COVID-19 Pandemic*, https://doi.org/10.1007/978-3-031-30844-4_1

exist, it was impossible to ascertain the true spread of infections; as a result, initial mortality estimates were very high.

Vaccines were developed extraordinarily fast, though that still took a full year, with the first mass vaccine roll-outs in December 2020–January 2021. The novelty of the disease and the initial expectation of its devastating impact on the population (Pueyo 2020) created a unique circumstance where, on the one hand, urgent public health interventions were required and, on the other hand, there were no readily available medical means to provide effective interventions. Around the globe, the first year of the pandemic, 2020, was the period when nonmedical interventions (NMIs) constituted the main defense against the disease. While defense by immunity was in the works in research labs, defense by government action seemed necessary (Ajana 2021), and the political incumbents in every country and locale found themselves in an unusual spotlight. They became doctors to the public.

What we call NMIs are in fact the modifications of individual behaviors as mandated by government. They are restrictions imposed on the actions of individuals in a society, with the aim of limiting behaviors that lead to virus spread. As such, NMIs are a classical example of public goods. Examples are lockdowns, business closures, and bans on events and gatherings. To protect the public, NMI policies were enacted by political incumbents around the world. When vaccines and new drugs and treatment protocols were developed and became available, NMIs continued to be used by many governments and to varying degrees remain in place in many of those countries as of this writing in fall 2022.

Despite the synchronicity of the threat and all governments' initially similar helplessness in the face of the virus, how governments acted to address the problem differed greatly across the world. To put it plainly, governments chose different NMIs, and some largely refrained from enacting any at all (Jasanoff et al. 2021). There was also substantial variation in the speed of their responses to the new threat, even when we account for the timing of initial virus detection in the various countries. Importantly, the stringency of the enacted NMIs – protective policies – varied considerably as well. Arguably, these differences at least partially determined the variation in health outcomes in the countries' populations (Daher-Nashif 2022; Kukovic 2022; McMann and Tisch 2021; Shvetsova et al. 2022a, b; Strand et al. 2022).

1.2 This Volume

As we take stock of the various aspects of the history of the COVID-19 pandemic, one important lesson to be learned concerns government behavior. Did some governments perform better than others? Were there any predictable or explainable shortcomings in their crisis responses? Will governments and countries that underperformed in this crisis fall short in other crises where responsible leadership might be required? The contributors to this volume compare and contrast what governments around the world did and did not do to stop the COVID-19 pandemic. To the rapidly expanding literature on lessons from the pandemic for the politics of crisis (e.g., Hale 2022; Lipscy 2020; van der Ven and Sun 2021) this volume adds the prism of political institutional influence on government policy response.

The theoretical framework that unifies the contributions in this volume is that the adoption of public health policies to mitigate the spread of the COVID-19 virus was a risky task for political incumbents (Flores and Smith 2013; Healy and Malhotra 2009). On the one hand, it was clear that COVID-19 posed a serious health threat. If a country did not adopt mitigation policies, COVID-19 could spread rapidly through that country's population, which could lead to high case and death rates and overwhelm the country's health infrastructure. But mitigation policies meant restrictive mandates on the population and businesses and carried heavy economic costs: a dramatic slowing of economic activity, reduced or negative growth, an increase in unemployment, and, potentially, a drastic economic restructuring.

As policymakers weighed the health benefits and economic costs of their mitigation policies, they took into account how the policies they adopted (or failed to adopt) would affect their prospects in future elections or even their very survival in office (Carey 2009; Powell 2000; Strom 2004). Regardless of how policymakers balanced health outcomes and economic outcomes during this period, they risked heavy personal political costs (Achen and Bartels 2004; Leon 2012; Heersink, Peterson, and Jenkins 2017). If they skillfully navigated the challenges presented by the pandemic, voters would likely reward them, but if they handled the situation poorly, voters would likely punish them – heavily (Malhotra and Kuo 2008).

Facing an urgent need to balance health outcomes, economic outcomes, and their own election prospects, elected officials carefully considered which policies to adopt or not adopt. As they mulled over their choices, they also considered what other policymakers were doing at the same time. Strategically, if an official wanted to avoid taking on the responsibility and costs of addressing the situation with the virus, they could have pushed the burden of dealing with the pandemic to other policymakers who also had the authority to adopt the needed measures (Weaver 1986; Zahariadis et al. 2020). This created patterns of intergovernmental task sharing in pandemic management that were a consequence of the strategic behaviors of national and subnational political incumbents (Benz and Sonnicksen 2017). The resulting balance of responsibilities in the pandemic varied greatly from country to country.

Institutional design, the formal rules in place that underlie the patterns of authority and accountability, provide a somewhat satisfactory statistical explanation for this country-specific balance of policymaking (Shvetsova et al. 2020). Characteristics such as regime type, federalism (Gasula et al. 2022), parliamentarism, condition of the political party system, executive ideology, and the timing and rules of upcoming elections all biased the patterns of policymaking during this period (Greer et al. 2020, 2021; Shvetsova et al. 2021).

Our authors offer evidence that there were patterns of similar behavior among the governments that shared institutional or political similarities. The literature has suggested some such patterns. Decentralization and duplication in policy authority can lead to a more efficient response than tight policy centralization (Iversen and Barbier 2021, Troisi and Alfano 2021, Shvetsova et al. 2020, 2021). There is also an emerging strand of literature on the potentially long-lasting institutional changes brought on by the political imperatives and opportunities which arose while mounting the pandemic response (Ladi and Wolff 2021).

Our authors also emphasize, however, that much of the political strategy in a crisis depends not on broad institution-based incentives but on the immediate political context and expediency, creating what appear to be the idiosyncrasies of individual country cases. Other potential determinants in incumbents' strategy choices in the pandemic included such factors as the state of economies (Celi et al. 2020), the preexisting tensions in political and social discourse (Benoit and Hay 2022), the timing of crisis onset relative to the phase in the national political process (Shvetsova et al. 2020), and the political and policy path dependence (Easton et al. 2022). The combination of such multiple factors made each country's circumstances truly unique; thus, the strategic environments faced by political incumbents differed in important ways, even if their institutional environments were similar.

As our contributors in this volume explore country comparisons, they delve into the political mechanisms that accounted for the biases in countries' pandemic responses and offer an integrated picture of how both general and unique influences combined to affect the policy strategies of incumbents. While some politicians behaved similarly to their close counterparts in other countries and, thus, fit generalizable patterns, others had to act under unique and pressing circumstances that were unrelated to the pandemic, and their resulting behaviors therefore defy general trends. Our authors here discern these systemic as well as idiosyncratic incentives that led to the varied choices of NMI strategies in their carefully constructed country narratives. Most of the contributors rely on the mixed-method approach, combining statistical analysis and analytical narratives.

A number of reliable data sources have emerged in the last few years reporting on NMI adoption throughout the world in response to the COVID-19 pandemic. Two of them, Protective Policy Index (PPI) (Shvetsova et al. 2022c) and Oxford COVID-19 Government Response Tracker (Hale et al. 2020), notably focus on the overall stringency of entire sets of policies that were put in place at any given point in time. Usefully, they also separate achieved stringencies by the levels of government issuing the policies. Contributors to this volume use both these datasets to evaluate governments' efforts in combating the pandemic. Many contributors here use the PPI dataset. Some of the authors and the editor contributed to the construction of the PPI dataset throughout 2020–2022 as members of the Binghamton University COVID-19 Policy Response Lab. Because the PPI data are so frequently used here, in order to save space in other chapters, in the next section, I describe the fundamentals of the PPI dataset, while the full data descriptor and free download information can be found in Shvetsova et al. (2022c).

The chapters that follow draw lessons from the small n comparisons and both narrate the handling of the health emergency by governments in select countries and propose theoretical explanations for incumbents' different approaches to an initially similar crisis.

Heller et al. (2023, Chap. 2 in this volume) observe in the European context that even as the professional public health advice became increasingly cohesive over time, the policy differences separating the countries did not significantly diminish. They attribute this phenomenon to the varying patterns of electoral vulnerability of ruling parties to the possible blame assignment for COVID-related policies. Specifically, in a complex theoretical argument, they suggest and demonstrate that stronger societal roots enabled governing parties to act more decisively when it came to adopting stringent public health measures to protect the population.

Focusing on South Asia, Adeel and Zhirnov (2023, Chap. 4) show that, despite the similarities in prepandemic conditions in India, Pakistan, and Bangladesh and their structural characteristics, the politics of response to the COVID-19 pandemic significantly diverged across these countries. The authors show how different, sometimes unexpected actors and channels became involved in public health decision-making. They point out the theoretical significance of institutional path dependence in epidemic response and the importance of congruence between the institutional legacies and current public health frameworks.

While earlier studies claimed that federations on the whole were more successful in mounting early pandemic policy responses than nonfederations, VanDusky-Allen (2023, Chap. 3) argues in her chapter that some federations were less successful than others. Specifically, she demonstrates that Latin American federations varied in the extent and effectiveness of their national-subnational coproduction of public health policies. She examines how a number of economic and political conditions at the national and subnational levels in each country that existed immediately prior to the pandemic influenced the willingness of both the national and subnational governments to adopt strict mitigation measures. She demonstrates how a combination of lagging economic development and populist national leadership resulted in reduced policy stringency in Brazil and Mexico compared to Argentina. The condition of the party system in Brazil and Mexico also resulted in a diminished role of the federal government (see also da Fonseca 2021). An important contrast that requires further exploration is that the subnational responsiveness in Mexico is correlated with the level of epidemiological threat, but in Brazil it is solely explainable by the partisanship of the governor.

Bayrali's chapter (2023, Chap. 5) compares the national-subnational dynamics of public health policymaking during the pandemic in Nigeria and South Africa. He demonstrates that, in Nigeria, the burden of responsibility for the unpopular pandemic restrictions was pushed off onto the subnational political incumbents, with the national government essentially free-riding. Meanwhile, in South Africa, the central government assumed political responsibility for the restrictive and unpopular public health policies. Bayrali's explanation for the variation in the patterns of task sharing

1 WHAT THE WORLD HAS LEARNED ABOUT THEIR GOVERNMENTS... 7

lies in the condition of the two countries' party systems. Linked electoral fates of subnational and national incumbents in South Africa made it advantageous for the national executive to shoulder the burden of unpopular policies.

Zhao (2023, Chap. 6) compares the strategies of the central governments in Malaysia and Indonesia in the introduction of NMIs and argues that the short-term political incentives served to create a positive push for political incumbents to ramp up measures, while the structural characteristics, primarily the condition of the labor force, served as binding constraints on the introduction of the more restrictive NMIs.

Bayar and Seyis (2023, Chap. 7) tackle the question of what influenced populist leaders in setting the direction of pandemic public health policies. Focusing on populist heads of state, the authors present the puzzle of populists' different reliance on science and experts in addressing the pandemic. While Bolsonaro in Brazil and Trump in the United States took a firm antiscience stance, Netanyahu in Israel and Erdogan in Turkey came across as very strongly proscience. Bayar and Seyis argue that populists' approaches to the pandemic and the way they behaved toward experts and scientists were thoroughly opportunistic. Populist leaders responded to two sets of influences: the ideology and beliefs of their core constituency and the specific contextual constraints in their countries at that particular moment, which affected the political costs of public health measures.

Chu's chapter (2023, Chap. 8) offers an analysis of the NMI strategies of the populist executives of Visegrad countries (Czech Republic, Hungary, Poland, and Slovakia). He argues that the Visegrad Four (V4) had the institutional capacity for a competent and speedy pandemic mitigation response. Whether the stringent NMIs were imposed or not crucially depended on public opinion and not on any personal beliefs and prejudices of the populist leaders. Chu demonstrates this by contrasting the different policy strategies in spring 2020 (supportive public) versus fall 2020 (changed constituent sentiment).

Catalano and Chan (2023, Chap. 9), in a novel contribution, identify a pattern of realism in judicial decision- making with regard to restrictive public health policies during the pandemic. The courts of last resort in Common Law systems in countries with British settler-colonial legacies have consistently refrained from overturning restrictive policies that governments enacted to control the impact of the pandemic. Furthermore, these authors show that, where the court stood in ideological opposition to the national executive, the court took the extra step of affirming the executive's policy (thereby going beyond refusing cert), possibly with the aim of reducing the ambiguity in the public's mind and of easing the continued implementation of the protective policy. That said, opinions accompanying such rulings were explicitly written to lower their precedential value beyond the parameters of the current crisis.

The concluding chapter, by Shvetsova and Zhirnov (2023, Chap. 10), summarizes the collective findings of the contributors in this volume and sketches a broader picture of discernible general trends in public health policy responses to the COVID-19 pandemic by governments worldwide.

1.3 Protective Public Health Policy Index (PPI)

Scholars almost never have the opportunity to compare the behaviors of many different governments in a similar or the same event and, thus, to discern, in an almost experimental fashion, how institutional and societal factors influence government decisions. The onset of the COVID-19 pandemic presented scholars with just such a rare opportunity. Rich or poor, all countries were equally lacking in appropriate medical solutions, and all were similarly under a threat from the infection, which was either already ravaging their countries or about to arrive there, imminently and inevitably. The adverse global event created a unique controlled experiment that made it possible to evaluate the impact of government characteristics on the policy effort that it devoted to managing the population-threatening crisis.

Political scientists have long been collating various characteristics of governments around the world. Measurements of government policy performance, however, are harder to make. The difficulty lies in constructing a measure that would capture the same meaning across different national contexts. Since our focus here is on the policy effort of incumbent governments in supplying their constituents with protective public health policies, indicators of the policy effort of incumbents are the NMIs that they put in place, and those differ by type and stringency. The PPI is a summary indicator, or rather a set of indicators, calculated on the basis of the original dataset (Protective Policy Index dataset) of such adopted NMIs and their srtingencies (Shvetsova et al. 2022c).

In the PPI dataset, incumbents' crisis responsiveness is captured by such variables as which actors respond, who responds first, how stringent (decisive) the issued NMI responses are, and the timing and stringency of actors' combined response. The PPI captures such aspects of *responsiveness* as the *timing* and *stringency* of public health policies since these NMIs were adopted and announced, and it is calculated separately for every *geographic unit* and *originating level of government*. The basic unit of analysis in the PPI data is *unit-day-level*. The stringency of the policy response is conceptualized in the PPI dataset as a calculated index across 15 categories of NMI policies (Appendix A, Tables A.1 and A.2). The index is calculated daily and separately for just those policies made at the level of a subnational unit, *Regional PPI* (e.g., just by the State of New York), just the policies made at the national level as they applied to a particular subnational unit, *National PPI* (e.g., just federal policies as they applied to the State of New York), and *Total PPI*, using whatever was the strictest restriction in that subnational unit – either national or subnational – in each category (again, e.g., for the State of New York). Because the weights of individual NMI categories in the calculation of PPIs are assigned by their authors and so are based on their assumptions, the dataset reports indices calculated by two alternative methods and additionally reports all index components for users to apply their preferred component weights or to include in their analyses separately. One of this volume's chapters, for example, uses individual PPI components in its data analysis (Bayar and Seyis 2023).

Frequently used in this volume are the country-level aggregates of the PPIs – averages of each of these three indexes across subnational units (weighed by population shares of the units in the country total). These indices capture protection via the NMIs of an average resident of a subnational unit due to 1) the policy efforts of regional governments (daily *Average Regional PPI*); 2) the national government (*Average National PPI*); and 3) from the combined efforts of governments at both levels (*Average Total PPI*).

Note that the PPI dataset does not contain data on implementation and compliance, but see Adeel and Zhirnov (2023), Barbalat and Franck (2022), Daoust et al. (2022), Jehn and Zajacova (2020), and Lazarus et al. (2020) for some global comparisons.

1.4 An Early Glimpse at the Global Variation in Policy Responses

As a prelude to the analyses in the chapters that follow, we will touch briefly on the issue of how governments around the world acted differently in the similar circumstances of the pandemic onset. While in later stages of the pandemic the selective availability of vaccines and treatments separated the rich from the poor and vaccine producers from vaccine buyers, in the onset period (Centers for Disease Control and Prevention 2016), the playing field was as leveled as ever across the globe. Furthermore, such were the initial assessments of the COVID-19 destructive power (Pueyo 2020) that the concerns were grave regardless of whether the virus had arrived in one's country or was only about to show up. In other words, from the perspective of protecting the population, the need for NMIs was nearly universal.

Governments' responsiveness was not uniform. The timing and stringency of NMI adoption varied significantly, and the load of policymaking borne by governments of different levels in introducing these policies also differed. Figure 1.1 illustrates this variation, and the chapters that follow all seek to explain the differences in policy responses. Histograms in Figure 1.1 report policy stringencies (the horizontal axis), as they were achieved on April 30, 2020, via the joint efforts of national and subnational governments (Average Total, left panels), just national government

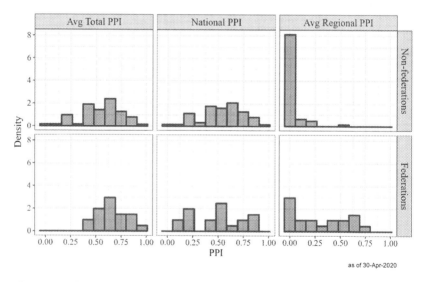

Fig. 1.1 Global variation in policy responsiveness during pandemic onset stage by level of government and by federal versus unitary type of government, on April 30, 2020. (Source: Shvetsova et al. (2022c))

efforts (Average National, middle panels), and just subnational government efforts (Average Regional, right panels), with a further breakdown between federations (bottom panels) and nonfederations (top panels). All panels except Average Regional policy stringencies in nonfederations show substantial variation. Notice in the left panes that the total NMI stringency in federations does not dip below 0.3, whereas among the nonfederations, there is no lower bound on NMI adoption.

Notice also that most of the policy effort in nonfederations is attributable to the national governments (compare top middle and top right panels). In federations, in contrast, both national and subnational governments on average were similarly active, though their relative involvement varied considerably (middle and right panels in bottom row). National policy stringency in federations was almost bimodally distributed; it was either low or relatively high. But when it came to Total PPI, the combination of NMIs adopted between the two levels of government ensured that the overall stringency (Average Total PPI) was unimodally distributed and at generally high levels.

The observed variation in the stringency of policy response by different governments to a similar threat is a puzzle that requires explanations of a political nature. This is the task we set for ourselves in this volume.

REFERENCES

Achen, C. H., & Bartels, L. M., 2004. *Blind retrospection: Electoral responses to drought, flu, and shark attacks*. Estudio/Working Paper 2004/199.

Adeel, A.B., & Zhirnov, A. (2023). COVID-19 response in India, Pakistan, and Bangladesh: Shared history, different processes. In O. Shvetsova (Ed.), *Political institutions and governments' behavior in pandemic mitigation: Year 2020 around the world* (pp. ...). Springer Nature

Ajana, B., 2021. Immunitarianism: defence and sacrifice in the politics of Covid-19. *History and philosophy of the life sciences, 43*(1), pp.1–31.

Bayar, M.C., Seyis, D. (2023). Populist responses to COVID-19: The cases of Turkey and Israel as examples of pro-science populism and the cases of the United States and Brazil as examples of science-skeptic populism. In O. Shvetsova (Ed.), *Political institutions and governments' behavior in pandemic mitigation: Year 2020 around the world* (pp. ...). Springer Nature

Bayrali, O.G. (2023). Center-regional political risk sharing in COVID-19 public health crisis: Nigeria and South Africa. In O. Shvetsova (Ed.), *Political institutions and governments' behavior in pandemic mitigation: Year 2020 around the world* (pp. ...). Springer Nature

12   O. SHVETSOVA

Benoît, C. and Hay, C., 2022. The antinomies of sovereigntism, statism and liberalism in European democratic responses to the COVID-19 crisis: a comparison of Britain and France. *Comparative European Politics*, pp.1–21.

Benz, A. and Sonnicksen, J. 2017. "Patterns of federal democracy: tensions, friction, or balance between two government dimensions." *European Political Science Review*, 9(1): 3–25.

Carey. J.M. 2009. *Legislative Voting and Accountability*. Cambridge: Cambridge University Press.

Catalano, M., Chan, A. (2023). Common law systems and COVID-19 policy response: protective public health policy in the United States, Canada, New Zealand, and Australia. In O. Shvetsova (Ed.), *Political institutions and governments' behavior in pandemic mitigation: Year 2020 around the world* (pp. …). Springer Nature

Centers for Disease Control and Prevention, 2016. "The Continuum of Pandemic Phase." National Center for Immunization and Respiratory Diseases (NCIRD), https://www.cdc.gov/flu/pandemic-resources/planning-preparedness/global-planning.html.

Chu, H. (2023). The Visegrad populist leaders' responses to the pandemic in 2020. In O. Shvetsova (Ed.), *Political institutions and governments' behavior in pandemic mitigation: Year 2020 around the world* (pp. …). Springer Nature

Daher-Nashif, S., 2022. In sickness and in health: The politics of public health and their implications during the COVID-19 pandemic. *Sociology Compass*, 16(1), p.e12949.

Daoust, J.F., Bélanger, É., Dassonneville, R., Lachapelle, E. and Nadeau, R., 2022. Is the Unequal COVID–19 Burden in Canada Due to Unequal Levels of Citizen Discipline across Provinces?. *Canadian Public Policy*, 48(1), pp.124–143.

Easton, M., De Paepe, J., Evans, P., Head, B., and Yarnold, J., 2022. Embedding expertise for policy responses to COVID-19: comparing decision-making structures in two federal democracies. *Public Organization Review*

Flores, A. Q., & Smith, A., 2013. Leader survival and natural disasters. *British Journal of Political Science*, 43(4): 821–843.

da Fonseca, E.M., Shadlen, K.C. and Bastos, F.I., 2021. The politics of COVID-19 vaccination in middle-income countries: Lessons from Brazil. *Social Science & Medicine*, 281, p.114093.

Gasulla, Ó., Bel, G. and Mazaira-Font, F.A., 2022. Ideology, political polarisation and agility of policy responses: was weak executive federalism a curse or a blessing for COVID-19 management in the USA?. *Cambridge Journal of Regions, Economy and Society*.

Greer, S.L., King, E.J., da Fonseca, E.M. and Peralta-Santos, A., 2020. The comparative politics of COVID-19: The need to understand government responses. *Global public health*, 15(9), pp.1413–1416.

1 WHAT THE WORLD HAS LEARNED ABOUT THEIR GOVERNMENTS... 13

Greer, S.L., King, E., Massard da Fonseca, E. and Peralta-Santos, A., 2021. *Coronavirus politics: The comparative politics and policy of COVID-19* (p. 663).

Hale, T., Webster, S., Petherick, A., Phillips, T., and Kira, B., 2020. Oxford COVID-19 Government Response Tracker, Blavatnik School of Government. Available at https://covidtracker.bsg.ox.ac.uk/

Hale, Thomas, et al. "What have we learned from tracking every government policy on COVID-19 for the past two years." BSG Research Note (2022).

Healy, A., and Malhotra, N., 2009. Myopic voters and natural disaster policy. *American Political Science Review*, 103(3): 387–406.

Heersink, B., Peterson, B. D., and Jenkins, J. A., 2017. Disasters and elections: Estimating the net effect of damage and relief in historical perspective. *Political Analysis*, 25(2): 260–268

Heller, W.B., Muftuoglu, E., Rosenberg, D. (2023). The institutional underpinnings of policy-making in the face of the COVID-19 pandemic in Europe. In O. Shvetsova (Ed.), *Political institutions and governments' behavior in pandemic mitigation: Year 2020 around the world* (pp. ...). Springer Nature

Hsiang, S., Allen, D., Annan-Phan, S. et al., 2020. The effect of large-scale anticontagion policies on the COVID-19 pandemic. *Nature*. https://doi.org/10.1038/s41586-020-2404-8

Iverson, T. and Barbier, E., 2021. National and sub-national social distancing responses to COVID-19. *Economies*, 9(2), p.69.

Jasanoff, S., Hilgartner, S., Hurlbut, J.B., Ozgode, O. and Rayzberg, M., 2021. Comparative Covid response: crisis, knowledge, politics. *Ithaca: CompCoRe Network, Cornell University*

Kukovič, S., 2022. How Novel Coronavirus has Shaken Public Trust in Decision-Making Institutions: Comparative Analysis of Selected European Union Members. Journal of Comparative Politics, 15(1), pp.9–19.

Ladi, S. and Wolff, S., 2021. The EU Institutional Architecture in the Covid-19 Response: Coordinative Europeanization in Times of Permanent Emergency. *Journal of Common Market Studies.*

León, S., 2012. How do citizens attribute responsibility in multilevel states? Learning, biases and asymmetric federalism. Evidence from Spain. *Electoral Studies* 31(1):120–130.

Lipscy, P.Y., 2020. COVID-19 and the Politics of Crisis. *International Organization*, 74(S1), pp.E98–E127.

Malhotra, N., and Kuo, A. G., 2008. Attributing blame: The public's response to Hurricane Katrina. *The Journal of Politics*, 70(1): 120–135.

McMann, K.M. and Tisch, D., 2021. Democratic regimes and epidemic deaths. *V-Dem Working Paper, 126.*

Powell, G. Bingham (2000). Elections as Instruments of Democracy. Majoritarian and Proportional Visions. New Haven: Yale University Press.

Pueyo, T., 2020. "Coronavirus: Why you must act now. Politicians, community leaders and business leaders: what should you do and when." *Medium*. March 10, 2020. https://medium.com/@tomaspueyo/coronavirus-act-today-or-people-will-die-f4d3d9cd99ca

Shvetsova, Olga; Zhirnov, Andrei; VanDusky-Allen, Julie; Adeel, Abdul Basit; Catalano, Michael; Catalano, Olivia; Giannelli, Frank; Muftuoglu, Ezgi; Riggs, Tara; Sezgin, Mehmet Halit; Tahir, Naveed; Zhao, Tianyi. 2020. *Journal of Political Institutions and Political Economy*. Vol. 1: No. 4, pp 585–613. https://doi.org/10.1561/113.00000023

Shvetsova, O., VanDusky-Allen, J., Zhirnov, A., Adeel, A.B., Catalano, M., Catalano, O., Giannelli, F., Muftuoglu, E., Rosenberg, D., Sezgin, M.H. and Zhao, T., 2021. Federal Institutions and Strategic Policy Responses to COVID-19 Pandemic. *Frontiers in Political Science*, 3, p.66.

Shvetsova, O., Zhirnov, A., Giannelli, F.R., Catalano, M.A. and Catalano, O., 2022a. Governor's party, policies, and COVID-19 outcomes: further evidence of an effect. *American Journal of Preventive Medicine*, 62(3), pp.433–437.

Shvetsova, O., Zhirnov, A., Giannelli, F., Catalano, M. and Catalano, O., 2022b. Can Correlation Between Governor's Party and COVID-19 Morbidity Be Explained by the Differences in COVID-19 Mitigation Policies in the States?. *American Journal of Preventive Medicine*, 62(6), pp.e381–e383.

Shvetsova, O., Zhirnov, A., Adeel, A.B., Bayar, M.C., Bayrali, O.G., Catalano, M., Catalano, O., Chu, H., Giannelli, F., Muftuoglu, E. and Rosenberg, D., 2022c. Protective Policy Index (PPI) global dataset of origins and stringency of COVID 19 mitigation policies. *Scientific Data*, 9(1), p.319.

Strand, M.A., Shyllon, O., Hohman, A., Jansen, R.J., Sidhu, S. and McDonough, S., 2022. Evaluating the Association of Face Covering Mandates on COVID-19 Severity by State. *Journal of Primary Care & Community Health*, 13, p.21501319221086720.

Strøm, K. Parliamentary Democracy and Delegation. In Eds. Kaare Strøm, K., Muller, W.C. & Bergman, T. *Delegation and Accountability in Parliamentary Democracies.* Oxford: Oxford University Press. 55–106. (2004).

Troisi, R. and Alfano, G., 2021. Is regional emergency management key to containing COVID-19? A comparison between the regional Italian models of Emilia-Romagna and Veneto. *International Journal of Public Sector Management*.

Van der Ven, Hamish, and Yixian Sun. "Varieties of crises: Comparing the politics of COVID-19 and climate change." *Global Environmental Politics* 21.1 (2021): 13–22.

VanDusky-Allen, J. (2023). An Analysis of Government Responses to COVID-19 in Latin America's Three Federations. In O. Shvetsova (Ed.), *Political institutions and governments' behavior in pandemic mitigation: Year 2020 around the world* (pp. ...). Springer Nature

Weaver, R.K. 1986. "The politics of blame avoidance. *Journal of public policy* 6(4), pp.371–398.

Zahariadis, N., Petridou, E. and Oztig, L.I., 2020. Claiming credit and avoiding blame: political accountability in Greek and Turkish responses to the COVID-19 crisis. *European Policy Analysis*, 6(2), pp.159–169.

Zhao, T. (2023). Pick your poison: Political expediencies, economic necessities, and COVID-19 response in Malaysia and Indonesia. In O. Shvetsova (Ed.), *Political institutions and governments' behavior in pandemic mitigation: Year 2020 around the world* (pp. ...). Springer Nature

CHAPTER 2

The Institutional Underpinnings of Policymaking in the Face of the COVID-19 Pandemic in Europe

William B. Heller, Ezgi Muftuoglu, and Dina Rosenberg

2.1 Introduction

As of this writing (July 2022), the novel coronavirus (COVID-19) pandemic has already taken the lives of over 6.6 million people (World Health Organization [WHO]). Although it appears to be subsiding or at least less deadly, the pandemic has pushed governments around the world to design and implement timely anti-COVID measures in the face of uncertainty about many aspects of the disease, its spread, and its treatment. Additionally, despite the fact that all governments were dealing with the same strain of the disease for the first eight months of the pandemic, until the more

---

W. B. Heller (✉) • E. Muftuoglu
Department of Political Science, Binghamton University, Binghamton, NY, USA
e-mail: wheller@binghamton.edu; emuftuo1@binghamton.edu

D. Rosenberg
Center on Democratic Performance, Binghamton University,
Binghamton, NY, USA
e-mail: dbalala1@binghamton.edu

© The Author(s), under exclusive license to Springer Nature
Switzerland AG 2023
O. Shvetsova (ed.), *Government Responses to the COVID-19 Pandemic*, https://doi.org/10.1007/978-3-031-30844-4_2

deadly "alpha" strain was discovered in the UK in September 2020 (Walker et al. 2021), government responses and outcomes varied dramatically across countries.

The first confirmed COVID-19 cases in Europe were reported in France on 24 January 2020 (WHO 2020). Germany and Finland reported cases of their own only a few days later, and data from the Johns Hopkins Coronavirus Research Center indicate that European Union countries with confirmed cases increased from six[1] at the beginning of February to fully sixteen[2] by the end of the month. By 19 March, when Lithuania saw its first confirmed case, the COVID-19 pandemic had a foothold in every country in the EU. Notwithstanding the rapid spread of the disease and the fact that all governments had access to the same information with respect to how best to respond to it, country responses differed widely in both approach and efficacy. For instance, on 1 March 2020 excess mortality from all causes was negative in every country in the European Union; by the end of that month, that statistic was up to nearly 140 percent in Spain and 90 percent in Italy, followed by Belgium and the Netherlands at nearly 45 percent and 0 in Denmark and Slovakia (Our World in Data 2022; see also Spiteri et al. 2020).

The reasons for differences in how the COVID-19 pandemic affects countries assuredly are many, ranging from country- and time- dependent factors such as tourism rates, population density, the status-quo allocation of health-care resources (Cox 2014), or the ideological complexion of government to such elements of institutional design as territorial organization (Shvetsova et al. 2020, 2021; Adeel et al. 2020), veto players (Tsebelis 1995), electoral rules (e.g., Iversen and Soskice 2006), and party systems (Budge and McDonald 2007; Iversen and Soskice 2006).

In this paper we propose a more nuanced explanation for why European countries significantly differ in their responses to the same disease by focusing on the partisan structure of the cabinet, specifically, the number of parties and their competitive context. As we see it, the number of parties in cabinet and their competitive relationship (Pavlović and Xefteris 2020)—i.e., whether and how they face off at the ballot box—should be an important consideration in analyzing government responses to crises like the current pandemic. The conventional common-pool resources

---

[1] Finland, France, Germany, Italy, Spain, and Sweden.
[2] Austria, Belgium, Croatia, Denmark, Estonia, Finland, France, Germany, Greece, Ireland, Luxembourg, Netherlands, Romania, Spain, and Sweden.

2 THE INSTITUTIONAL UNDERPINNINGS OF POLICYMAKING IN THE FACE... 19

logic would suggest that the quality of government action should decline with the number of parties in government, as parties either try to shift blame or claim credit for policy. We build on Pavlović and Xefteris (2020) in arguing that the common-pool logic works differently in politics than economics in that it should be influenced by interparty electoral competition: parties that don't compete for the same voters have no direct electoral reason to compete on policy either.

The core of our argument is that the less parties compete for what Pavlović and Xefteris (2020) term "impressionable" voters, the less they need worry about claiming credit or shifting blame for policy benefits or costs that fall on voters. By this token, in a two-party majority coalition, each of the parties will in general represent a broader swathe of constituents than the average party in a majority coalition with three or more members. Consequently, whereas small parties with limited constituencies are relatively free to focus on their target voters rather than seeking to attract more marginal voters, larger parties do not have that luxury and will focus on "impressionable" voters. One tactic for stealing away other parties' voters (and retaining one's own) involves taking credit for successes and assigning blame for failures. Armed with the "winner-takes-all" logic inherent in two-party competition versus the more cooperative "consociational" logic of multiparty competition (Lijphart 1969), one could argue that competition between two players raises the electoral stakes and impedes decision-making. Thus, we argue that the effect of the number of parties within ruling coalitions upon policies is nonlinear: both single-party governments and multiparty coalitions, all else being equal, are expected to outperform two-party coalitions. We then take the argument a step farther, observing that to the extent that the ministerial structure of cabinet government parses out distinct, nonoverlapping jurisdictions (Shepsle 1979), parties should have incentives to produce the best policies they can because there is no one else to share the blame or take the credit.[3]

We explore the viability of our argument by applying it to four cases from the European Union—Denmark, Finland, Spain, and Italy—chosen for their multiparty legislatures and mix of cabinet types (number of parties, majority/minority). All four countries we examine share some basic similarities. They are constitutionally unitary parliamentary regimes with

---

[3] This part of our argument depends on the maintained hypothesis that politicians (and ministers in particular) *believe* some nontrivial number of voters is able to connect policies to ministries and their ministers.

decentralized healthcare systems, and they all have multiparty legislatures with nine or more parties and an effective number of parliamentary parties greater than four. They differ widely in the type of cabinet and number of parties in the coalition, from one in Denmark's minority cabinet, to two major parties within Italian and Spanish coalition governments, to five in Finland's majority coalition, as well as the relative sizes and legislative weights of cabinet parties.

This chapter is organized as follows. In the next section we briefly describe the logic of coalition policymaking under the classic model of coalition formation and explain why the model in its original form fails to explain policymaking during crises. In the following section, we present our main theoretical argument, where we introduce two important concepts—partisan competitive relationships and the compartmentalization of policy responsibilities—and demonstrate how this addition to the model enriches its explanatory power. After that we provide empirical evidence by tracing anti-COVID policymaking in the selected four country cases. Finally, we discuss our results and present conclusions.

2.2 The Classic Model of Coalition Policymaking and Why It Does Not Work in Times of Crisis

The conventional wisdom holds that ministers make and implement policy (see Alexiadou 2016), and while their counterparts in other ministries might raise a public eyebrow from time to time (in multiparty governments, that is; in single-party governments, disagreements should be worked out *in camera* under the watchful eye of the party leader and according to established party decision-making procedure; cf. Bagehot 1873), the empirical regularity of collective cabinet responsibility, whereby ministers support their counterparts, generally obtains. Public disagreements should be minor or primarily for show (Fortunato 2019; Sagarzazu and Klüver 2017) once the boundaries of coalition policy and policymaking have been set, whether that is achieved through detailed coalition agreements (Bäck et al. 2017) or the careful allocation of ministries and ministerial jurisdictions (Dewan and Hortala-Vallve 2011; Laver and Shepsle 1996).

The portfolio-allocation model of coalition formation (Laver and Shepsle 1996) essentially equates coalition formation and coalition policy positioning. The naïve model can be criticized for setting up a massive, multiparty logroll, which in turn opens the door to the common-pool problems discussed earlier. The naïve model, moreover, runs up against the question of whether coalition parties would be willing to give free rein to their partners in light of the possibility that unexpected issues might arise to make ministerial autonomy at best unpalatable (Riker 1980).

One straightforward guarantee that coalition partners won't go too far out of line is the *de facto* veto every coalition partner has over coalition survival and any concomitant policymaking (Tsebelis 1995). Other common steps to ensure that unforeseen policy concerns don't hand too much power to coalition partners include coalition agreements (Bäck et al. 2017), carving out central coordinating authority for the finance minister (Alexiadou and Gunaydin 2019), or portfolio design and allocation (e.g., Dewan and Hortala-Vallve 2011; Heller 2001). Whatever the method, however, the effect is to constrain ministerial autonomy.

Ministers acting under constraints might be desirable in the normal course of day-to-day policymaking. In a crisis that demands rapid and perhaps even bold action, however, those same constraints could be crippling. At the same time, a crisis should usefully undermine these constraints. First, the emergence of new issues and concerns leaves the usual jurisdictional lines blurred and faded, rendering moot existing divisions of authority so that the correspondence between coalition formation and coalition policy that follows from the Laver and Shepsle (1996) portfolio-allocation model no longer holds. Second, the subsequent intracoalition negotiations to define crisis-specific jurisdictions and jurisdictional authorities should seek to build a decision-making structure specific to the problem at hand. It might take some time to get the details right, possibly leading to a delayed policy response vis-à-vis single-party governments, but once they do settle on a division of authority, multiparty coalitions then should function well.

2.3   Theoretical Argument

In the normal give-and-take of everyday politics, as discussed earlier, government policymakers rule over their jurisdictions within the constraints of coalition agreements (Bäck et al. 2017), party hierarchies, or strategic considerations. There should in equilibrium be no real *behavioral* differences between majority and minority or multiparty and single-party governments, as all government decision makers go about their business within their respective jurisdictions. We argue that in times of crisis such as the onset of the COVID-19 pandemic the aforementioned equilibrium expectations no longer apply, which leads us to the hypothesis that the differences between cabinet types should yield observably and predictably different outcomes. We present our theoretical argument in what follows, which brings to the forefront (1) the number of parties in the cabinet and (2) the nature of electoral competition (for instance, whether the parties compete for the same voters or not).

The number of parties in government should matter primarily for several reasons. First, from the common-pool resource perspective, any value attached to policy, positive *or negative*, should create problems. For policies that parties want to claim credit for, the problem is classic: as long as they can take all or most of the credit and corresponding electoral benefit for policy measures while shouldering only a fraction of the blame for consequences (such as increased debt or taxes), they should ratchet up spending. And the division of policymaking into jurisdictions controlled by coalition parties facilitates precisely the kind of jurisdiction-specific credit claiming that leads to such problems. If the potential fallout from policymaking is unpredictable or possibly even negative, as in the case of imposing restrictions on movement and gatherings along with mandates such as mask wearing and vaccination restrictions, the possibility that credit for any benefits will be shared with other coalition partners while the responsible party will bear the brunt of voter anger should mean that necessary policies will be undersupplied (Olson 1965). In either case, for policies voters like as well as for policies they don't, the more parties there are in the governing coalition, the more difficult it is expected to be for government to supply good public policy.

There is more to cabinet policymaking than the tragedy of the commons, however. Parties' incentives to compete on policy grounds ought to depend at least in part on the extent to which they compete for the same voters ("impressionable" voters; Pavlović and Xefteris 2020). For example, regional parties that don't run candidates against each other really don't compete electorally at all and thus have no reason to compete on policy (or any other) grounds. Viewed from this perspective, the common pool problem takes on a different hue: single-party governments, of course, have no coalition partners to compete with and cannot suffer any potential pernicious collective-action effects. Two-party governments, by contrast, should work very differently from multiparty governments, all else being equal.

2 THE INSTITUTIONAL UNDERPINNINGS OF POLICYMAKING IN THE FACE... 23

Single-party majority governments, as noted, should for their part be able to make and implement their preferred policies fairly straightforwardly. But what about minority governments? On one hand, it seems reasonable to suppose that minority-government policies that can be passed only with outside support should involve more compromises and be less effective overall than what majority governments produce. This view makes sense in particular for the kinds of policies parties might want to claim credit for. Alternatively, however, inasmuch as the need for value tradeoffs in policy means that policies involve costs as well as—if not more than—benefits, nongovernment parties might be happy to support measures they see as necessary even as they let the government bear the costs.

In many respects, including perhaps an expectation of delayed response to crises relative to single-party governments, two-party and multiparty governments should be similar. But in other respects, we think two parties in a coalition should look very different from three or more parties. Parties in multiparty governments are able to appeal to different sets of voters because, realistically, they have relatively limited constituencies. The more parties in government, the fewer jurisdictions any given party is likely to control.[4] And if specific jurisdictions are of interest to specific constituencies, the fewer jurisdictions parties control, the less reason they have to compete for uncommitted voters. In general, the same is less likely to be true of parties in two-party (majority) governments, where party constituencies must be on average larger.[5] The larger a party is, the more likely it

---

[4] Whatever coalition policy looks like in terms of bills passed—whether policies are the product of some overall interparty compromise, as the mass of coalition scholarship assumes (e.g., Tsebelis and Money 1997), or are parsed out to parties in line with the cabinet portfolios they control (e.g., Alexiadou and Hoepfner 2019; Heller 2001; Laver and Shepsle 1996)—actual bills are elaborated and policies implemented in whichever ministries have jurisdiction.

[5] It is, of course, possible that two-party coalitions will form parties that will not seek to attract the same sets of uncommitted voters. Grand coalitions might be an example of this, at least inasmuch as the parties in question compete for voters more with other parties closer to their own positions than with each other. Or, for instance, the case of Giuseppe Conte's second government, a coalition of the populist Movimento 5 Stelle and the antipopulist Partito Democratico, which apparently disagreed not only on questions of policy but on fundamental questions of the proper conduct of politics. As Horowitz (2019) reported, "the joining of two parties that have called each other every name in the book, including Mafiosi and kidnappers, internet trolls and hatemongers, was remarkable." We expect, given that they start from a position of political and almost existential conflict, that such coalitions should be able to achieve little.

is to be a so-called catch-all party that seeks to attract support from multiple and varied constituencies; and while smaller parties partnered with larger parties in two-party coalitions might themselves have small, clearly identifiable constituencies, the same is less likely to be true of their coalition partners. As a consequence, the larger parties in such coalitions have an incentive to use credit claiming and blame shifting to try to poach voters from their partners, and the smaller partner parties have no choice but to respond in kind.

In sum, we have argued that, while the classic common-pool logic might hold up for straightforward economic policymaking, we believe there are good reasons to think we might observe something different where the policy tradeoffs are qualitatively different. Indeed, we think a health crisis like the COVID-19 pandemic represents just such a crisis. Rather than government failures following from common-pool problems, we expect multiparty coalition governments to perform better than their two-party brethren, all else being equal. The empirical evidence presented in the next section corroborates this hypothesis.

2.4   CASE SELECTION

Italy, Spain, Finland, and Denmark are similar in some—but not all—important respects. At the macro level, all are multiparty parliamentary democracies with decentralized healthcare systems; they entered the pandemic in more or less similar circumstances with respect to healthcare resources. For instance, all four countries have similar numbers of physicians and hospital beds per capita (Table 2.1), though the Nordic countries have nearly twice as many nurses per 100,000 inhabitants as their southern counterparts. With respect to health spending, there are notable differences between the southern and northern countries, depending on the metric used (Table 2.2): spending as a percentage of GDP is roughly equal across cases, but a sizeable gap opens up between Denmark and Finland on the one hand and Spain and Italy on the other, depending on whether spending is measured in terms of per-capita purchasing power, euros per capita, or total spending in euros.

Figure 2.1 shows a snapshot of confirmed cases of COVID-19 in our four countries over the first six months of the pandemic. We focus here on the first six months because we are interested in the rapidity and effectiveness of initial government responses, and we highlight the number of cases rather than deaths (though deaths and cases do covary) because the

Table 2.1 Physicians, nurses, and hospital beds per 100,000 inhabitants in Denmark, Finland, Italy, and Spain

Country	Physicians[a]	Nurses[d]	Hospital beds[d]
Denmark	400.1[b]	1009.9	243
Finland	348.0[c]	1022.8[c]	361
Italy	425.1	574.2	314.1
Spain	457.7	586.9	297.2

Eurostat (2022a, b, c, Table 1)

[a]2020

[b]2019 data

[c]2018 data

[d]2018

[e]2014 data

Table 2.2 Healthcare spending in Denmark, Finland, Italy, and Spain, 2019

Country	Euros	Euros	Purchasing Power Standards (PPS)	Percentage of GDP (%)
		per inhabitant		
Denmark	31137	5355	3915	9.96
Finland	21992	5042	3258	9.15
Spain	113674	2412	2573	9.13
Italy	155249	2599	2611	8.67

Eurostat (2021), Table 2.1

relevant policies—e.g., lockdowns, mask mandates, restrictions on business and private (and public) gatherings—are directed not at treating the disease per se but rather at containing its spread. As can be seen, Italy and Spain—particularly Spain—were hard hit by the disease in the early days (a pattern that repeated in the fall 2020 wave until Denmark surpassed both in early 2021). Finland's rolling seven-day count of confirmed cases never exceeded double digits throughout the first year of the pandemic.

Clearly, some of the differences across our cases could be due to structural or contextual factors beyond government control. The populations of Italy and Spain, for example, were over eight times larger than those of Denmark and Finland in 2020 (World Bank 2020a), though Spain, Italy,

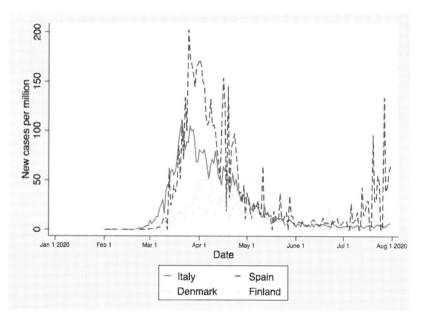

Fig. 2.1 Daily new COVID-19 cases per million residents in Denmark, Finland, Italy, and Spain. (Source: Mathieu E et al. (2020) Coronavirus Pandemic (COVID-19). Our World in Data, Oxford. https://ourworldindata.org/coronavirus)

and Denmark were fairly close in terms of population density (World Bank 2020b). But Spain and Italy are far more popular as tourist destinations, for example, which could easily have impacted the number of cases early on. In addition, all four countries exhibited the familiar wave pattern that characterizes this and other pandemics we have seen. That said, however, we suspect that at least some of the dramatic differences in the incidence of COVID-19 across these cases can be traced to the dynamics of cabinet policymaking.

From a political-institutional perspective, all four countries we examine share some basic similarities. They are unitary parliamentary regimes with decentralized healthcare systems, and all have multiparty legislatures with nine or more parties and an effective number of parliamentary parties greater than four (Table 2.3). They nevertheless show variation in the type of cabinets and number of parties, with a single-party minority cabinet in

2 THE INSTITUTIONAL UNDERPINNINGS OF POLICYMAKING IN THE FACE... 27

Table 2.3 Parliamentary and cabinet parties in Denmark, Finland, Italy, and Spain

Country	Legislative parties[a]	ENPP[b]	Total seats[a]	Large[a]	Small[a,d]	Cabinet parties[c]	Basis	Diff 1[e]	Diff2[f]
Denmark	11	5.9	179	47	6	1	Minority	0.268	0.268
Finland	10	6.4	200	49	5	5	Majority	0.045	0.100
Italy	12	4.3	630	227	1	4	Majority	0.183	0.360
Spain	13	4.75	350	123	1	3	Minority	0.243	0.343

[a]Regional representatives not elected on a party list (i.e., from the Faroe Islands and Greenland for Denmark, from Åland for Finland, and from the Val d'Aosta and expatriate voters for Italy) are counted as if from a single, distinct party (Parties and Elections in Europe 2022)
[b]Effective number of parliamentary parties (Casal Bértoa 2022)
[c]The count for Italy incudes two small splinter parties that have not competed in elections, and the count for Spain includes one member of the Communist Party (PCE) that ran on a joint ticket with Podemos (Casal Bértoa 2022)
[d]Not including representatives not affiliated with a party
[e]Difference in legislative seat shares of the largest and second largest parties in cabinet
[f]Difference in legislative seat shares of largest and third largest parties in cabinet

Denmark, multiparty coalition government in Finland, and two major-party coalition governments in Italy and Spain).

In both Finland and Denmark, the seat share of the largest parliamentary party is close to 25 percent, while in neither country does any party have less than 2.5 percent of seats. In Spain and Italy, by contrast, the largest party in each country holds about 35 percent of seats, while the smallest party's seat share is less than half a percent. In Spain and Italy, the second largest party has only about half as many seats as the largest, compared to 90 and 98 percent in Denmark and Finland, respectively.

As can be seen in Fig. 2.2, Spain and Italy both eventually adopted fairly strong measures to deal with the COVID-19 pandemic. To account for the cumulative policy stringency, we make use of the average total Protective Policy Index (Shvetsova et al. 2022). The index consists of 15 nonmedical interventions (e.g., border closures, school closures, restriction on businesses, required social distancing and self-isolation) and takes into account policy efforts at both national and subnational levels. Relative to the number of cases and deaths, however, both countries probably should have done more and sooner. Italy's response was essentially a slow ratcheting-up of policy stringency that began in a timely fashion but then

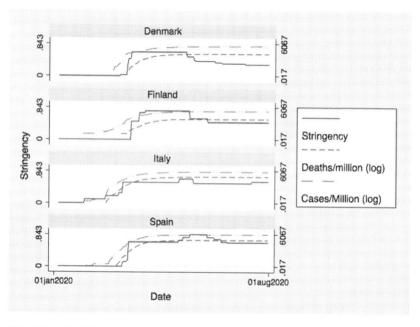

Fig. 2.2 Covid impact and early responses in Denmark, Finland, Italy, and Spain: stringency and timing. (Source for stringency: Shvetsova et al. 2022; source for Deaths/million and Cases/million: Mathieu E et al. (2020) Coronavirus Pandemic (COVID-19). Our World in Data, Oxford. https://ourworldindata.org/coronavirus)

lagged as cases and deaths increased rapidly. Spain also applied measures of increasing stringency over time but also took longer to do anything in the first place. That both initially reacted more quickly than Finland and Denmark might reasonably be attributed to the negotiating costs of allocating new and unforeseen responsibilities to ministries (for Finland) and, for Denmark, where the government's parliamentary basis was just over 26 percent, the need to get a solid parliamentary majority behind the government's efforts. The key point, to reiterate, is that we see Finland's (and Denmark's) aggressive response in the face of a much lower impact of the disease as at least partly a consequence of coalition dynamics. We delve into this argument in the case studies that follow.

2.5 Spain and Italy

There are several explanations in the literature for why the Italian and Spanish responses to COVID-19 in the first wave were so chaotic, delayed, and close to failure. One obvious problem lay in the fact that both countries, Italy in particular, were guinea pigs in fighting COVID-19 in Europe. Both countries were already in a full-on war against the pandemic well before it had become clear what clinical practices (e.g., who should be hospitalized and how to treat the disease) and other policy interventions (including testing systems, masking, social distancing, and isolation) would be most successful. Timing aside, many observers highlight structural issues, including underinvestment in universal healthcare provision, especially following the 2008 world financial crisis and subsequent austerity measures (e.g., Stuckler et al. 2017; Casula and Pazos-Vidal 2021); high population density (Gutiérrez et al. 2020); and demography, with Italy being the most aged country in the EU with 23 percent of the population aged 65 or more) and Spain also harboring a large elderly population (17 percent; Dowd et al. 2020).

Apart from the timing and structural factors, many researchers emphasize the role of political institutions, political culture, and governance, especially the mechanism of coordination between the center and regions in crisis management (Casula and Pazos-Vidal 2021; Parrado and Galli 2021; Peralta-Santos et al. 2021; Ruiu 2020; Malandrino and Demichelis 2020; Mattei and Del Pino 2021). Center-regional relations are of paramount importance in both Italy and Spain, which are unitary by constitution but share several quasi-federal arrangements and—importantly for the handling of the pandemic—healthcare federalism. Most authors argue that inefficient center-regional coordination coupled with criticism from regional parties, both ruling and opposition, as well as blame-shifting games between center and regions are responsible for the delay in response in both countries, though more so in Spain. Deficits in state capacity represent another powerful explanation for the first-wave policy failures (Bosancianu et al. 2020; Capano 2020).

The following section takes the form of a series of analytic narratives outlining the main policy responses in Italy and Spain and applying our theoretical perspective highlighting partisan and coalitional dynamics to each case. It is important to note that we view our theory as consistent with and complementary to existing explanations and not as a strict alternative. By the conventional wisdom on coalition policymaking, which builds on common-pool logic, Spain's and Italy's two-party coalitions should perform better than Finland's five-party cabinet, and Denmark's single-party government should do better still, all else being equal. But as the data on the spread of COVID-19 in the early days of the pandemic show, Finland fared better than all three other countries, and the spread of the disease in both Denmark and Finland was much less pronounced than in Italy and Spain. This observation runs contrary to the conventional wisdom but is consistent with our claim that that the number of parties within ruling coalitions has a nonlinear effect on policies: both single- and multiparty coalitions, all else equal, are expected to outperform two-party coalitions.

2.6   ITALY

After Italy confirmed its first COVID-19 case in January 2020, then-Prime Minister Conte immediately announced the appointment of a special commissioner for the COVID-19 emergency. Even so, it was more than three weeks before the first quarantine zones were declared in Northern Italy. Beginning on 22 February, as the situation deteriorated, the Italian government adopted what on paper appeared to be the strictest set of measures in Europe to slow down the spread of the virus. For instance, all sports events were suspended, as were the Carnival of Venice and the Carnival of Ivrea, and quarantine zones were declared in several regions. Measures included closure of schools, universities, cultural, and other public venues, bans on social gatherings, and suspension of commercial activities. The scope of the lockdown was unprecedented in the context of peacetime democratic Europe (Bull 2021). However, because time was of utmost importance in the face of the virus's exponential spread, the government's dilatory response had drastic consequences, especially in the Northern regions.

In early and mid-March, the government extended lockdowns to incorporate new affected areas in the North, which led to people migrating to the South to escape restrictions, often in the overcrowded transport that could add to the already rising number of cases. Roberto Speranza, Minister of Health at the time of the start of the pandemic and the only member of the Free and Equal parliamentary group to hold a ministerial portfolio, distinguished himself from his coalition partners by his hawkish calls for a full lockdown. It is important to note here that Speranza's electoral concerns probably were quite different from those of the larger coalition parties.[6] As such, it was fortunate that he held the health portfolio, where he was free to impose within the powers of his ministry such measures as he saw fit. Conte and the other ministers, primarily concerned with the state of the economy, initially took milder stances.

Finally, on 21 March, after realizing that partial lockdowns did not work as intended and amid fears that the healthcare system in poorer Southern regions was not prepared to cope with its own population, let alone migrants from the North, Conte's government introduced a full lockdown. People were required to stay at home, many commercial businesses were closed, but by that time the health infrastructure was overloaded, and daily deaths had already reached an all-time high. The lockdown was extended in early April, when all "nonessential" business activity was suspended and fines were increased for noncompliance. Cases finally began to decline in May to early June 2020, which allowed the government to lift certain measures (e.g., reopening businesses and recreational activities and resuming first interregional and then international travel). During the summer the government acted decisively (reinstating measures where they were appropriate and lifting them where they were deemed unnecessary), and the public generally complied. By fall 2020 Italy had shaken off the image of a country that drastically failed its response to COVID-19 (Bull 2021). In addition, during the pandemic's second wave in fall 2020, Italy fared better than many other European countries, which some researchers (e.g., Bontempi 2021) attributed to specific policy measures, such as masking in public and teleworking, which helped reduce interactions among people, along with strict enforcement and high public compliance.

According to our argument, Italy's inefficient and weak initial response is at least in part due to the composition of the coalition government—primarily two major parties with a few ministries held by minor partners—in which parties competed for voters and thus were incentivized to engage in blame shifting and credit claiming. When the pandemic struck, Italy was led by the Conte II cabinet, formed in September 2019 as a majority coalition between the big-tent populist Five-Stars Movement (M5S) and

---

[6] Parliamentary groups in Italy often are unrelated to electoral parties. Free and Equal won fourteen list seats in the 2018 Camera dei Diputati election as an electoral coalition, but had disbanded as an electoral contender by the 2019 European Parliament elections. We assume that its minister, Roberto Speranza, thus was essentially an independent insofar as electoral politics were concerned. And it is difficult as of this writing to gauge Italia Viva's current electoral interests, as it has yet to contest elections.

center-left Democratic Party (PD), with three independent ministers and one minister from the Free and Equal parliamentary group (Camara dei Diputati; Casal Bertoa 2022). Shortly after the government was formed, two of its ministers left the PD as part of a small schism party, Italia Viva (IV), but remained in the coalition.

The ruling center-left coalition in Italy emerged from ideologically incompatible parties in 2019 in the wake of a major government crisis in which the Lega left the ruling center-right coalition. Thus, the government already was highly fragmented and polarized when the pandemic hit. On the one hand, the ruling M5S is a centrist, populist, catch-all party that has been described as anti-establishment, Eurosceptic, and antiglobalist. Its support comes primarily from the eastern and more rural parts of the country (Russo et al. 2017). On the other hand, the junior coalition partner, PD, is a pro-European, progressive, left-Christian party. They share little common ground with respect to policy, a division that extends to how they characterize each other as well (e.g., Horowitz 2019)

Disagreements between coalition partners are partially to blame for hampering the policy measures adopted to combat COVID-19. For example, even before the first confirmed case of COVID-19, the parliamentary parties had several large disputes over pandemic-related spending, which ultimately resulted in IV's leaving the ruling coalition (albeit much later, in January 2021) and provoked a government crisis (BBC News 2020a, b). By April, with the number of new cases dropping rapidly, the public rallied behind its government. The prime minister's ratings soared, and he did not hesitate to claim credit for managing the crisis. Defending his plans to slowly lift what was Europe's longest-running lockdown amid criticism from the business community and politicians in the opposition and ruling coalitions alike, Conte declared that "if I could turn back the clock, I'd do it all again" (Aljazeera 2020b). During the first wave of the COVID-19 pandemic, many parliamentary opposition members as well as representatives of regional governments objected to pandemic-related restrictions (Bosa et al. 2021), so for Conte it was an easy victory.

2.7   Spain

The early response to the pandemic in Spain was quite similar to that in Italy. Spain's first case of COVID-19 was confirmed on 1 February 2020 (Johns Hopkins Coronavirus Research Center). And despite lockdowns in several neighborhoods on 7 March, 120,000 people participated in the International Women's Day march, which international health authorities were quick to criticize the next day. By 12 March, all regional governments had closed schools and some travel restrictions had been introduced. But it was not until a month and half later, after the detection of the first case, that Sánchez's government announced a state of alarm from 15 March, which included partial lockdown and then the first full lockdown (28 March–12 April). After 15 March, nonessential movement was limited and nonessential businesses and schools were closed. By then COVID-19 had already penetrated into all provinces of the country, and in several regions the number of infections was growing exponentially. The second lockdown (starting 28 March) saw a tightening of previous restrictions, forcing all nonessential employees to work from home. The state of alarm allowing emergency restrictions was extended five times and lasted until 20 June, each time receiving less and less support from the parliament and thus forcing the government to adopt milder anti-COVID-19 measures. The relaxation of confinement measures was predicated on the establishment of four phases, which allowed regionally tailored policymaking on the bases of key indicators (local transmission rates and healthcare capacity). The strategy for exiting from the lockdown regime presumed mandatory mask wearing, restrictions on social gatherings, remote work if possible, and maintaining social distancing (Dubin 2021).

As our theory suggests, inefficiencies in the Spanish response to COVID-19 during the first wave could be traced back to the structure of the governing coalition, within which two major parties (or, more accurately, one major party and one rising new party with ambitions to take its place) reluctantly reached a consensus. The first coalition government in Spain since before Franco took control of the country in the 1930s formed just before the first confirmed case of COVID-19 in the country. Pedro Sánchez of the Socialist Workers' Party (PSOE) formed a two-party minority government (21 seats shy of the 176 seats required for a majority) with Unidos Podemos (UP). Not only was the country shaken by the deep political and government crises over the preceding year, but the freshly baked coalition partners-in-government had no time to adjust to a coalition governing style and learn to cooperate with each other, let alone prepare to fight a global pandemic. Although from a strict left-right ideological perspective the PSOE and UP were much closer to each other in policy terms than their Italian counterparts, including with respect to dealing with the pandemic, they also developed—and publicly aired—important disagreements on many fronts beyond just pandemic response early on.

Indeed, Sánchez's cabinet during the pandemic was even more polarized, hostile, and fragmented than Conte's in Italy. First, to reiterate, Sanchez's government was a minority coalition, with only 155 out of 350 seats in the Congreso de Diputados. The situation was similar in the upper chamber, where the governing parties controlled only 115 of 256 seats. More importantly for our argument, both coalitions were highly fractious, with partner parties publicly engaging in blame-shifting games as well as publicly disagreeing on subjects ranging from "monarchies to rappers" (Hedgecoe 2021) the judiciary, or regional policy. As we see it, the governing parties' conflictual relationship—in a very real sense, UP was a new, upstart party that had only entered parliament in 2015 and was actively seeking to annex the political space long held by the PSOE—is fundamental to understanding why Spain's initial response was so ineffectual.

2.8   DENMARK AND FINLAND

Perhaps the most common explanation in the literature for Finland's and Denmark's successes with respect to COVID-19 early on is Nordic exceptionalism. This perspective, highlighting the Nordic countries' characteristic high trust in government leading to high compliance with government policy mandates, is consistent with explanations that tout as well-established institutions existing governing features, media support, and Nordic culture.

Policymakers in both Finland and Denmark took their cues from expert opinions and closely followed the recommendations of their national healthcare agencies (Christensen et al. 2022). In Finland, this meant relying on the advice of the Finnish Institute for Health and Welfare, which was established in the 1960s and 1970s to provide systematic knowledge in health care (Moisio 2020). For its part, the Danish government first established an emergency crisis response coordination commission made up of members of various national authorities (Saunes et al. 2022). Additionally, in early May, Denmark formed a new agency under the Ministry of Justice to ensure coronavirus preparedness.

Building on their own public-health institutions, Nordic countries already had a foundation for cooperating with each other in sharing information and knowledge. Rules established under the Nordic Public Health

Preparedness Agreement, signed in 2002 by Denmark, Finland, Iceland, Sweden, and Norway to ensure cooperation and assistance for emergencies like COVID-19, required the signatories to exchange experiences, to share information on planned measures (including legislative initiatives), and to provide opportunities for cooperation. Given the strong basis for cooperation and utilization of expertise, Denmark's and Finland's initial success in dealing with COVID-19 seemed unsurprising (Saunes et al. 2022; Socialstyrelsen). That said, however, our theoretical framework provides additional understanding of what it is that makes the Nordics different.

In what follows, we turn to an analysis of the Danish and Finnish responses to the first wave of the pandemic and apply our theoretical argument, which complements existing explanations in the literature. Where Spain and Italy both had two-party governments at the outset of the pandemic, Finland had a five-party majority coalition and Denmark a single-party minority cabinet with a government basis of only 27 percent of parliamentary seats. If policymaking and the consequent electoral implications of credit or blame allocation followed common-pool resource logic, neither country should have responded well to the COVID-19 threat. In Finland, the expected infighting among parties seeking to ensure that their connection to government policies would work to their own electoral advantage *at the expense of their coalition partners* should have made putting together an effective response to the disease difficult at best—leave aside the difficulties posed by transaction costs alone as coalition partners negotiate how to deal with an unforeseen crisis. Moreover, in Denmark, opposition parties could have made demands on the government that would have rendered any kind of coherent policymaking impossible. But they did not.

2.9 FINLAND

Sanna Marin of the Social Democratic Party of Finland (SDP) replaced Antti Rinne at the head of Finland's five-party governing coalition government in December 2019, not long before the first COVID-19 case in the country. The speed and scope of the government response to COVID-19 were perhaps surprising given that the center-left government, made up of Marin's SDP (40 seats), the Center Party (KESK, 31 seats), the Green League (VIHR, 20 seats), the Democratic Union|Left Alliance (VAS, 16 seats), and the Swedish People's Party (RKP-SFP, 9 seats), had formed only six months earlier as Finland's first coalition cabinet led from the left in twenty years.

Finland's first confirmed case of COVID-19 came early in the pandemic, when a tourist from Wuhan, China, was diagnosed with the illness on 29 January (Tiirinki et al. 2020, p. 649). The disease did not really get going in the country until March, however, with the total number of reported cases going from three on 25 February to ten on 2 March and then to forty-four just a week later (Johns Hopkins Coronavirus Research Center). The first death came on 7 March. On 16 March, at a press conference attended by all coalition party leaders except Green League leader Maria Ohisalo (who was duly present at another press conference the next day), the government declared a state of emergency, closed K-12 schools and universities, banned public gatherings of more than ten people, closed museums, cultural venues, and sports facilities, and initiated a two-week quarantine period for travelers from abroad. It was at the time arguably the strictest government response in Europe to the pandemic. Thereafter, Prime Minister Marin held daily press conferences with representatives of all coalition parties in attendance until 27 March, demonstrating a unified front and cooperation among governing partners. These conferences followed a narrative structure such that each minister's delivery continued from and built on the previous speaker's last point. This unified approach continued throughout the pandemic, passing its first major test with the passage on 25 March via emergency legislation of 118 measures, including restaurant closures and travel restrictions between the Helsinki metropolitan area and the rest of the country until after Easter (Koljonen and Palonen 2021). The force of this measure is noteworthy, in particular given Finns' penchant for taking advantage of the Easter holiday and the season's warming weather to travel north to enjoy the snow (Moisio 2020).

Superficially, one would expect the parties in Finland's government to have a hard time cooperating. Not only should the number of government parties make reaching agreement difficult, but they might be motivated to ensure that they don't lose votes to—and if possible that they gain votes from—their partner parties on the left. Nonetheless, Interior Minister Dr. Maria Ohisalo of the Green League emphasized that during a crisis like COVID-19, it is important that the leaders of the five coalition parties cooperate and act like one leader (Janjuha-Jivraj 2020). She described her approach to governmental cooperation during COVID-19 as a win-win-win—everybody needs to win something (Janjuha-Jivraj 2020), attributing Finland's effective response to existing trust and cooperation among coalition partners: "The strength of the pre-existing working relationships is critical in having created trust and a clear way of how to work together and reach effective decisions" (Janjuha-Jivraj 2020).

It makes sense that policymaking and implementation in response to a crisis like the COVID-19 pandemic would work best if line ministers can work together to create an effective response to the virus without destroying the economy. And in Finland, consistent with our argument about the advantages of minimizing jurisdictional overlap, crucial portfolios for COVID-19 policymaking were held by different coalition partners. Aside from the prime minister (SDP), the finance and economic affairs ministries fell to KESK, the education and health ministries were held by VAS, and VIHR controlled the interior ministry. Far from contributing to intracoalition division, we argue that this separation of responsibilities contributed to cabinet members' ability to work harmoniously to fight the virus. To reiterate, the less overlap there is across parties with respect to ministerial jurisdictions, the less parties have to worry about sharing either blame for other parties' missteps or credit for their successes. We believe that this motivates parties and their ministers both to design effective policy and to support their partners' efforts to do the same, which is in striking contrast to the interparty jealousies that seem to have dominated policymaking in Spain's and Italy's two-party governments.

We argue that multiparty coalitions are at an advantage in dealing with COVID-19 in part because more parties means less overlap in jurisdictional responsibilities. Evidence in line with this claim indicates that Finnish voters were willing and able to point fingers at specific agencies and ministers when it came to evaluating the government's COVID-19 response. For instance, many tweets criticized the Finnish Institute for Health and Welfare for not being strict enough, criticism that extended to the Ministry of Social Affairs and Health and to Minister Aino-Kaisa Pekonen of the Left Alliance; and while the entire government was not immune from blame, voters were clearly able to connect parties to their jurisdictional responsibilities (Koljonen and Palonen 2021). This aligns with our argument, as constituents distinguished among coalition parties and their portfolio responsibilities, obviating the utility of playing the credit-claiming or blame games when it comes to policy responsibility.

The government began to discuss plans for a gradual reopening in early May, deciding to move from large-scale restrictions to targeted measures focusing on a "test, trace, isolate and treat" strategy (European Observatory on Health Systems and Policies 2022). Beginning on 14

May, kindergarten and elementary schools were returned to normal, travel restrictions for Schengen countries were relaxed, and outdoor recreational facilities were reopened. In addition, from 1 June the ten-person limitation on social gatherings was increased to fifty, and dining at restaurants and sport facilities was allowed. While the country was not opening fast enough for some business sectors (the Confederation of Finnish Industries, businesses representatives, and economists criticized the government for the slow reopening), the center-right opposition in the parliament supported the government's careful and steady approach to lifting restrictions (Moisio 2020).

Finland nicely illustrates the advantages of promoting cooperation among coalition partners while at the same time clearly dividing up responsibilities. Government press conferences highlighted policy collaboration across ministerial portfolios, even as they gave individual ministers from the various coalition parties a platform to present plans for fighting COVID-19 in their jurisdictions. Since constituents could easily link the decisions taken in different jurisdictions to the coalition parties responsible for them, this helped to reduce credit claiming and blame shifting.

2.10 DENMARK

Denmark reported its first confirmed case of COVID-19 on 27 February, several weeks after the first Finnish case. Within only about two weeks, on 11 March, Prime Minister Mette Frederiksen announced strict measures that would take effect two days later (and three days before the first confirmed COVID-19 death in the country). The response was strict as well as rapid and included the closure of schools, recreational centers, cultural institutions, and libraries, required public employees to work from home, and shut down international borders. Finland's first death from the disease had come earlier, on 7 March, only a week before Denmark's (Johns Hopkins Coronavirus Research Center), but by 16 March Denmark's response to the pandemic joined that of Finland as one of the strictest in Europe.

Uniquely among our cases, Denmark's government was a single-party Social Democrat (SD) minority cabinet that had taken office under the leadership of Mette Frederiksen shortly after the June 2019 elections with parliamentary support from the Socialist People's Party (SF), the Red-Green Alliance (EL), and the Social Liberal Party (RV). The government had the full support of parliament at the onset of the pandemic, to the extent that it took parliament only twelve hours to pass major amendments to the Epidemic Act of Denmark, in force since 1915, on the same day that Frederiksen announced the closures (Herrmann 2020). The amendment passed, moreover, with unanimous parliamentary support.

The act passed on 12 March shifted power from regional authorities to the government. In this centralization of usually decentralized authorities, Denmark's actions were similar to those measures (de jure or de facto) in Spain and Italy, although compliance was arguably better. In normal times, regional epidemic commissions held the authority not only to prohibit events but also to initiate treatment without consent that would force individuals to isolate and hospitals to admit patients (Herrmann 2020). The act transferred these powers to the health minister, along with additional new authority to order the police to isolate, examine, and treat persons believed to be infected. And though the act raised questions among scholars about human rights violations, public trust in government remained high. According to a survey of government COVID-19 responses conducted in fourteen advanced democracies, 95 percent of Danish respondents thought that their government handled the pandemic well, the highest approval among all countries in the survey (Devlin, and Connaughton 2020)

The Danish government was controlled by a single party, but as a minority government with an actual government basis of only 48 of 179 parliamentary seats it could not govern alone or hope for strategic abstentions that might help it get its way. Rather, it had to cooperate from the outset with other parties and the societal interests they represented. In addition, like the partners in Finland's five-party coalition, the Social Democrats had every incentive to design the best policies they could as no other party could either steal the credit or share the blame for policies voters didn't like. This facilitated cooperation in parliament as well as with businesses and meant that the Danish government's response would be inclusive, informed, and effective.

Prime Minister Frederiksen announced plans at the end of March for gradually reopening the country beginning in mid-April. After three weeks of lockdown, Denmark was, with Austria, the first country in Europe to start reopening. Following consultations with the other parties in parliament, the reopening started with daycare centers and elementary schools, with the idea of helping to ease parents' childcare responsibilities and encourage the workforce to return to "normal." At a press conference, Frederiksen referred to the balance between healthcare and the economy, mentioning the possibility of a deep recession if the country remained in lockdown for too long and noting that "the situation we are in is far more complicated than appreciating human life." She added that "we cannot open a textbook—neither on healthcare nor economy—and find the right answer" and recognized that ultimately "the strategy we follow is a political choice" (Aljazeera 2020a).

Frederiksen's government balanced its stringent disease-fighting measures with new fiscal policies. Three days after the announcement of closures, the government put in effect a temporary wage compensation program to prevent businesses from firing their employees. The government also covered 75 percent of the wages of furloughed salaried workers (Ornston 2021), later announcing another program for self-employed workers. And, consistently with the minority government's need to make and maintain allies, Denmark's recovery package was based on a proposal by Denmark's largest trade union and employer organization (ILO 2020 as cited in Ornston 2021). Like Finland, the Danish government put cooperation front and center in its COVID-19 response, and for its efforts it was one of the most successful countries in terms of fighting the spread of the virus. The government might have had the institutional tools to manage the pandemic on its own, but the political calculations of minority governance were sufficient motivation for the government to maintain close cooperation with the opposition rather than dealing with the pandemic unilaterally.

2.11   Discussion

It is easy to look at our four cases and pass off their differences as predictable consequences of country-specific cultural distinctions or manifestations of the more general north-south divide. But to our eyes, these are not explanations but rather alternative ways of describing the observation that Spain and Italy are more similar to each other than to Denmark or Finland—and vice versa—in their COVID-19 responses. In arguing that the number and competitive relationships of parties in government is a basic driver of government behavior and response, we have offered a reasonable, theoretically grounded explanation for the quality, extent, and effectiveness of government action that is consistent with our cases. More broadly, we have suggested that thinking of government policymaking in terms of the standard common-pool resource problem is likely misguided.

We focus in this chapter on governments' initial response to the pandemic because we believe that the first reactions to something like the novel coronavirus are particularly telling. What happened later is, of course, partly attributable to what governments did at the outset, but it is possible as well that later waves were worse than they might otherwise have been because governments, buoyed by their initial successes, loosened the reins of control more or less quickly than they should have. What we find in our four case studies fits nicely with our theoretical outlook: where government parties had little reason to compete on COVID-19-response policy grounds, whether because party responsibility for specific measures was easily traceable or because the parties in question had little cause to seek to attract voters away from each other, the response went fairly smoothly. Where accountability was murkier (or parties had incentives to make it murky), due to both shared responsibilities and electoral competition, things were more problematic.

We do not, of course, claim that interparty coalition politics is the only determinant of government policymaking. Far from it. Other factors, from existing policy to the resources available for policymaking and implementation to opposition parties (Sartori 1976), surely matter a great deal. We do think coalition politics is important, however; what government does matters, and what government does is—or at least should be if elections and government formation, i.e., parliamentary democracy, mean anything—a consequence of the parties in government and their interactions.

This chapter represents a first stab at the broader idea that party competition is inconstant not only across time (Sagarzazu and Klüver 2017) but also across parties. We have presented case-study evidence that clearly delineating the policy responsibilities of parties in government might make it easier for them to cooperate, and we have argued that this is more easily done the more parties there are in government. A more comprehensive look at this notion would look at more cases and employ tools to more comprehensively nail down the relationship between number of parties in government and the degree to which they manage to cooperate. It is our hope this chapter will serve as a first step toward such research.

References

Adeel AB, Catalano M, Catalano O, Gibson G, Muftuoglu E, Riggs T, Sezgin MH, Shvetsova O, Tahir N, VanDusky-Allen J, Zhao T, Zhirnov A (2020) COVID-19 policy response and the rise of the sub-national governments. Canadian Public Policy, 46(4):565–584. https://doi.org/10.3138/cpp. 2020-101

Alexiadou D (2016) Ideologues, partisans, and loyalists. Oxford University Press, Oxford.

Alexiadou D, Gunaydin H (2019) Commitment or expertise? Technocratic appointments as political responses to economic crises. European Journal of Political Research 58(3): 845–865. https://doi.org/10.1111/1475-6765.12338

Alexiadou D, Hoepfner D (2019) Platforms, portfolios, policy: How audience costs affect social welfare policy in multiparty cabinets. Political Science Research and Methods 7(3): 393–409. https://doi.org/10.1017/psrm.2018.2

Aljazeera (2020a) Denmark prepares to ease coronavirus restrictions. https://www.aljazeera.com/economy/2020/4/3/denmark-prepares-to-ease-coronavirus-restrictions. Accessed 2 Aug 2022

Aljazeera (2020b) Conte defends 'slowly-slowly' lifting of Italy's lockdown. https://www.aljazeera.com/news/2020/4/28/conte-defends-slowly-slowly-lifting-of-italys-lockdown. Accessed 2 Aug 2022

Bäck H, Müller WC, Nyblade B (2017) Multiparty government and economic policy-making: Coalition agreements, prime ministerial power and spending in Western European Cabinets. Public Choice 170(1–2): 33–62. https://doi.org/10.1007/s11127-016-0373-0

Bagehot W (1873) The English constitution (2nd ed.). Little, Brown, and Company, Boston.

BBC News. (2020a). Italy political crisis erupts over EU Covid spending. https://www.bbc.com/news/world-europe-55661781. Accessed 2 Aug 2022

BBC News. (2020b). Italian PM Conte resigns in split over Covid response. https://www.bbc.com/news/world-europe-55802611. Accessed 2 Aug 2022

Bontempi E. (2021) The Europe second wave of COVID-19 infection and the Italy "strange" situation. Environmental Research 193:110476–110476. https://doi.org/10.1016/j.envres.2020.110476

Bosa I, Castelli A, Castelli M, Ciani O, Compagni A, Galizzi M M et al (2021) Corona-regionalism? Differences in regional responses to COVID-19 in Italy. Health Policy 125(9):1179–1187.

Bosancianu C M, Hilbig H, Humphreys M, Sampada KC, Lieber N, Scacco A (2020). Political and Social correlates of Covid-19 mortality. SocArXiv https://doi.org/10.31235/osf.io/ub3zd.

Budge I, McDonald M D (2007) Election and party system effects on policy representation: Bringing time into a comparative perspective. Electoral Studies 26(1): 168–179. https://doi.org/10.1016/j.electstud.2006.02.001

Bull M (2021) The Italian government response to Covid-19 and the making of prime minister. Contemporary Italian Politics 13(2): 149–165. https://doi.org/10.1080/23248823.2021.1914453

Camara dei Diputati (2022). http://www.camera.it. Accessed 11 July 2022

2 THE INSTITUTIONAL UNDERPINNINGS OF POLICYMAKING IN THE FACE... 43

Capano G (2020) Policy design and state capacity in the COVID-19 emergency in Italy: If you are not prepared for the (un)expected, you can be only what you already are. Policy & Society 39(3):326–344. https://doi.org/10.108 0/14494035.2020.1783790

Casal Bértoa F (2022) Database on WHO GOVERNS in Europe and beyond. PSGo. http://www.whogoverns.eu.

Casula M, Pazos-Vidal S (2021) Assessing the multi-level government response to the COVID-19 crisis: Italy and Spain compared. International Journal of Public Administration 44(11–12):994–1005. https://doi.org/10.1080/01900692.2021.1915330

Christensen T, Jensen MD, Kluth M, Kristinsson GH, Lynggaard K, Lægreid P, Niemikari R, Pierre J, Raunio T, Adolf Skúlason G (2022) The Nordic governments' responses to the Covid-19 pandemic: A comparative study of variation in governance arrangements and regulatory instruments. Regulation & Governance. https://doi.org/10.1111/rego.12497

Cox GW (2014) Reluctant democrats and their legislatures. In: Shane M, Saalfeld T, Strøm K (ed) Oxford Handbook of Legislative Studies. Oxford University Press, Oxford, p 696–717

Devlin K, Connaughton A (2020). Most approve of national response to COVID-19 in 14 advanced economies. Pew Research Center. https://www.pewresearch.org/global/2020/08/27/most-approve-of-national-response-to-covid-19-in-14-advanced-economies. Accessed 2 Aug 2022

Dewan T, Hortala-Vallve R (2011) The Three as of government formation: Appointment, allocation, and assignment. American Journal of Political Science 55(3):610–627. https://doi.org/10.1111/j.1540-5907.2011.00519.x

Dowd JB, Andriano L, Brazel DM, Rotondi V, Block P, Ding X, Liu Y, Mills MC, (2020) Demographic science aids in understanding the spread and fatality rates of COVID-19. Proceedings of the National Academy of Sciences 117(18):9696–9698. https://doi.org/10.1073/pnas.2004911117

Dubin KA (2021) Spain's response to COVID-19. In: Greer SL, King EJ, Fonseca EM, Peralta-Santos A (ed) Coronavirus Politics: The Comparative Politics and Policy of Covid-19. University of Michigan Press, Ann Arbor. https://doi.org/10.3998/mpub.11927713.

European Observatory on Health Systems and Policies. (2022, April 14) Country update: Monitoring and surveillance. https://eurohealthobservatory.who.int/monitors/hsrm/all-updates/hsrm/finland/monitoring-and-surveillance. Accessed 14 Nov 2022

Our World in Data (COVID-19) (2022) Excess mortality during the Coronavirus Pandemic. Our World in Data, Oxford. https://ourworldindata.org/excess-mortality-covid. Accessed 14 Nov 2022

Fortunato D (2019) Legislative review and party differentiation in coalition governments. The American Political Science Review 113(1):242–247. https://doi.org/10.1017/S000305541800062X

Gutiérrez E, Moral-Benito E, Oto-Peralías D, Ramos R (2020) The spatial distribution of population in Spain: An anomaly in European perspective, Banco de España working papers: 2028.

Healthcare expenditure statistics (2021) Eurostat, Luxembourg. https://ec.europa.eu/eurostat/statistics-explained/index.php?title=Healthcare_expenditure_statistics. Accessed 28 Jul 2022

Healthcare personnel statistics—beds (2022a) Eurostat, Luxembourg. https://ec.europa.eu/eurostat/statistics-explained/index.php?title=Healthcare_resource_statistics_-_beds. Accessed 28 Jul 2022

Healthcare personnel statistics—nursing and caring professionals (2022b) Eurostat, Luxembourg. https://ec.europa.eu/eurostat/statistics-explained/index.php?title=Healthcare_personnel_statistics_-_nursing_and_caring_professionals. Accessed 28 Jul 2022

Healthcare personnel statistics—physicians (2022c) Eurostat, Luxembourg. https://ec.europa.eu/eurostat/statistics-explained/index.php?title=Healthcare_personnel_statistics_-_physicians. Accessed 28 Jul 2022

Hedgecoe G (2021) Spain's governing partners show bad blood in public. Politico, Arlington. https://www.politico.eu/article/spain-government-coalition-bad-blood-psoe-podemos Accessed 2 Aug 2022

Heller WB (2001) Making policy stick: Why the government gets what it wants in multiparty parliaments. American Journal of Political Science 45(4):780–798. https://doi.org/10.2307/2669324

Horowitz J (2019) How Giuseppe Conte of Italy went from irrelevant to irreplaceable. The New York Times, NY. https://www.nytimes.com/2019/08/29/world/europe/italy-conte-government-salvini.html. Accessed 2 Aug 2022.

Iversen T, Soskice D (2006) Electoral institutions and the politics of coalitions: Why some democracies redistribute more than others. The American Political Science Review 100(2):165–181. https://doi.org/10.1017/S0003055 406062083

Janjuha-Jivraj S (2020) Finland's Maria Ohisalo: Navigation through Covid-19 requires leadership based on win-win approach. Forbes, Jersey City. https://www.forbes.com/sites/shaheenajanjuhajivrajeurope/2020/05/20/ohisalo-covid-19-finland/?sh=3f574cf52561

Johns Hopkins Coronavirus Research Center. https://coronavirus.jhu.edu. Accessed 2 Aug 2022

Koljonen J, Palonen E (2021) Performing COVID-19 control in Finland: Interpretative topic modelling and discourse theoretical reading of the government communication and hashtag landscape. Frontiers in Political Science 3. https://doi.org/10.3389/fpos.2021.689614

Laver M, Shepsle KA (1996) Making and breaking governments: cabinets and legislatures in parliamentary democracies. Cambridge University Press, Cambridge

Lijphart A (1969) Consociational democracy. World Politics 21(2): 207–225. https://doi.org/10.2307/2009820

Malandrino A, Demichelis E (2020) Conflict in decision making and variation in public administration outcomes in Italy during the COVID-19 crisis. European Policy Analysis 6(2): 138–146. https://doi.org/10.1002/epa2.1093.

Mathieu E, Ritchie H, Rodés-Guirao L, Appel C, Giattino C, Hasell J, Macdonald B, Dattani S, Beltekian D, Ortiz-Ospina E, Roser M (2020) Coronavirus Pandemic (COVID-19). Our World in Data, Oxford. https://ourworldindata.org/coronavirus. Accessed 3 Nov 2022

Mattei P, Del Pino E (2021) Coordination and health policy responses to the first wave of COVID-19 in Italy and Spain. Journal of Comparative Policy Analysis: Research and Practice 23(2): 274–281. https://doi.org/10.1080/1387698 8.2021.1878886

Moisio S (2020) State power and the COVID-19 pandemic: the case of Finland. Eurasian Geography and Economics 61(4–5):598–605. https://doi.org/1 0.1080/15387216.2020.1782241

Olson M (1965) The Logic of Collective Action: Public Goods and the Theory of Groups. Oxford University Press, Oxford

Ornston D (2021) Denmark's response to Covid-19: A participatory approach to policy innovation. In Greer SL, King EJ, De Fonseca EM, Peralta-Santos A (ed), Coronavirus politics: The comparative politics and policy of Covid-19. University of Michigan Press, Ann Arbor, p 249–263. https://doi.org/10.3998/mpub.11927713

Parrado S, Galli D (2021) Intergovernmental veto points in crisis management: Italy and Spain facing the COVID-19 pandemic. International Review of Administrative Sciences 87(3): 576–592. https://doi.org/10.1177/0020852320985925

Parties and Elections in Europe (2022) http://www.parties-and-elections.eu Accessed 28 Jul 2022

Pavlović D, Xefteris D (2020) Qualifying the common pool problem in government spending: the role of positional externalities. Constitutional Political Economy 31(4): 446–457. https://doi.org/10.1007/s10602-020-09306-6

Peralta-Santos A, Saboga-Nunes L, Magalhães PC (2021) A Tale of two pandemics in three countries Portugal, Spain, and Italy. In King EJ, Da Fonseca EM, Peralta-Santos A (ed) Coronavirus politics: The comparative politics and policy of COVID-19. University of Michigan Press, Ann Arbor

Riker WH (1980) Implications from the disequilibrium of majority rule for the study of institutions. American Political Science Review 74(2): 432–446. https://doi.org/10.2307/1960638

Herrmann, J Rothmar (2020) How Denmark's epidemic act was amended to respond to COVID-19. Bill of Health. https://blog.petrieflom.law.harvard.edu/2020/05/26/denmark-global-responses-covid19/. Accessed 3 Aug 2022

Ruiu ML (2020) Mismanagement of Covid-19: Lessons learned from Italy. Journal of Risk Research 23(7–8): 1007–1020. https://doi.org/10.108 0/13669877.2020.1758755

Russo L, Riera P, Verthé T (2017) Tracing the electorate of the MoVimento Cinque Stelle: an ecological inference analysis. Rivista Italiana Di Scienza Politica 47(1): 45–62. https://doi.org/10.1017/ipo.2016.22

Sagarzazu I, Klüver H (2017) Coalition governments and party competition: Political communication strategies of coalition parties. Political Science Research and Methods 5(2): 333–349. https://doi.org/10.1017/psrm.2015.56

Sartori G (1976) Parties and party systems: A framework for analysis. Cambridge University Press, Cambridge.

Saunes IS, Vrangbæk K, Byrkjeflot H, Jervelund SS, Birk HO, Tynkkynen LK, Keskimäki I, Sigurgeirsdóttir S, Janlöv N, Ramsberg J, Hernández-Quevedo C, Merkur S, Sagan A, Karanikolos M (2022) Nordic responses to Covid-19: Governance and policy measures in the early phases of the pandemic. Health policy 126(5): 418–426. https://doi.org/10.1016/j.healthpol.2021.08.011

Shepsle KA (1979) Institutional arrangements and equilibrium in multidimensional voting models. American Journal of Political Science 23(1): 27–59. https://doi.org/10.2307/2110770

Shvetsova O, Zhirnov A, VanDusky-Allen J, Adeel AB, Catalano M, Catalano O, Giannelli F, Muftuoglu E, Riggs T, Sezgin MH, Tahir N, Zhao T (2020) Institutional origins of protective COVID-19 public health policy responses: informational and authority redundancies and policy stringency. Journal of Political Institutions and Political Economy 1(4): 585–613. https://doi.org/10.1561/113.00000023

Shvetsova O, VanDusky-Allen J, Zhirnov A, Adeel AB, Catalano M, Catalano O, Giannelli F, Muftuoglu E, Rosenberg D, Sezgin MH, Zhao T (2021) Federal institutions and strategic policy responses to COVID-19 pandemic. Frontiers in Political Science 3. https://doi.org/10.3389/fpos.2021.631363

Shvetsova O, Zhirnov A, Adeel AB et al (2022) Protective Policy Index (PPI) global dataset of origins and stringency of COVID 19 mitigation policies. Sci Data 9, 319. https://doi.org/10.1038/s41597-022-01437-9

Socialstyrelsen. Nordic public health preparedness agreement. https://www.socialstyrelsen.se/globalassets/sharepoint-dokument/dokument-webb/ovrigt/nordiskt-halsoberedskapsavtal%2D%2D-engelska.pdf. Accessed 30 Oct 2022

Spiteri G, Fielding J, Diercke M, Campese C, Enouf V, Gaymard A, Bella A, Sognamiglio P, Sierra Moros MJ, Riutort AN, Demina YV, Mahieu R, Broas M, Bengnér M, Buda S, Schilling J, Filleul L, Lepoutre A, Saura C, Mailles A, … Ciancio BC (2020) First cases of coronavirus disease 2019 (COVID-19) in the WHO European Region, 24 January to 21 February 2020. Euro surveil-

2 THE INSTITUTIONAL UNDERPINNINGS OF POLICYMAKING IN THE FACE… 47

lance: bulletin Europeen sur les maladies transmissibles = European communicable disease bulletin 25(9): 2000178. https://doi.org/10.2807/1560-7917. ES.2020.25.9.2000178

Stuckler D, Reeves A, Loopstra R, Karanikolos M, McKee M (2017) Austerity and health: the impact in the UK and Europe. European Journal of Public Health, 27(suppl_4):18–21. https://doi.org/10.1093/eurpub/ckx167

Tiirinki H, Tynkkynen LK, Sovala M, Atkins S, Koivusalo M, Rautiainen P, Jormanainen V, Keskimäki I (2020) COVID-19 pandemic in Finland— Preliminary analysis on health system response and economic consequences. Health policy and technology 9(4): 649–662. https://doi.org/10.1016/j. hlpt.2020.08.005

Tsebelis G (1995) Decision making in political systems: veto players in presidentialism, parliamentarism, multicameralism and multipartyism. British Journal of Political Science 25(3): 289–325. https://doi.org/10.1017/S0007123 400007225

Tsebelis G, Money J (1997) Bicameralism. Cambridge University Press, Cambridge

Walker A, Vihta KD, Gethings O, Pritchard E, Jones J, House T, Bell I, Bell JI, Newton JN, Farrar J, Diamond I, Studley R, Rourke E, Hay J, Hopkins S, Crook D, Peto T, Matthews P C, Eyre DW, … Pouwels KB (2021) Tracking the emergence of SARS-CoV-2 Alpha Variant in the United Kingdom. New England Journal of Medicine 385(27): 2582–2585. https://doi.org/10.1056/ NEJMc2103227

World Bank (2020a) Population Data. World Bank, Washington DC. https:// data.worldbank.org/indicator/SP.POP.TOTL?end=2021&locations=DK-FI-IT-ES&start=2020. Accessed 1 Aug 2022

World Bank (2020b) Population Density Data. World Bank, Washington DC. https://data.worldbank.org/indicator/EN.POP.DNST?locations=EU-DK-IT-FI-ES. Accessed 1 Aug 2022

World Health Organization, Geneva. 2020. https://covid19.who.int/. Accessed 21 Nov 2022

CHAPTER 3

An Analysis of Government Responses to COVID-19 in Latin America's Three Federations

Julie VanDusky-Allen

3.1 Introduction

As COVID-19 spread quickly and aggressively throughout Latin America in early 2020, the World Health Organization (WHO) and other healthcare agencies advised governments to adopt a series of nonpharmaceutical intervention policies that could have helped them control the spread of COVID-19 within their borders. These policies varied in their level of stringency. Some policies only restricted the behavior of individuals who had the virus. Other policies placed blanket restrictions on all people regardless of their health status. While these policies would likely help governments reduce COVID-19 case and death rates, the willingness of governments in Latin America to adopt these policies varied greatly.

In this chapter I use the Protective Policy Index (PPI) to compare the stringency of government responses to COVID-19 in three Latin American

J. VanDusky-Allen (✉)
School of Public Service, Boise State University, Boise, ID, USA
e-mail: julievanduskyallen@boisestate.edu

© The Author(s), under exclusive license to Springer Nature Switzerland AG 2023
O. Shvetsova (ed.), *Government Responses to the COVID-19 Pandemic*, https://doi.org/10.1007/978-3-031-30844-4_3

49

countries: Argentina, Brazil, and Mexico. All countries are relatively comparable in terms of political development. They are all younger democracies, and they are all multiparty, presidential federations. Additionally, pandemic policymaking was predominately led by the executive branch within each country (at the national and/or subnational levels) (Lupien et al. 2021; Shvetsova et al. 2022). Yet the PPI, a measure of how stringent a country's COVID-19 policies were on a given day, demonstrates that each country took different approaches to the pandemic. Overall, Argentina adopted the most stringent measures throughout most of 2020, while Brazil and Mexico adopted less stringent policies.

In this chapter I analyze why Latin America's three federations took different approaches to the pandemic. I argue that since Argentina is the most developed country within the region and its governing party at the national level was the oldest and most well established, it was relatively easier for the government to adopt strict mitigation measures. I also argue that since the government usually plays an important role in healthcare provision within Argentina, it was relatively easy for the government to take on the role of addressing the pandemic as well. In contrast, I argue that Brazil and Mexico adopted less stringent measures overall because they were comparatively less developed, and they were led by populists at the national level.

Beyond examining the overall government response to COVID-19 in Argentina, Brazil, and Mexico, I also examine which levels of government contributed the most to each country's overall response. I find that in Argentina, the federal government played a dominant role in addressing the pandemic. In Brazil, states' responses dominated. In Mexico, both the federal government and state governments played a role in responding to the pandemic. I argue that the nature of the party system in Argentina made it easier for the federal government to lead the response to the pandemic, while the party systems in Brazil and Mexico made it harder.

Since states played an important role in responding to the pandemic in Mexico and Brazil, I also analyze factors that influenced state-level responses in these countries. I find that at the state level in Mexico, COVID-19 case rates had a positive effect on the stringency of measures, while poverty had a negative impact. In Brazil, only the partisanship of the governor could explain state-level responses.

In the next four sections I use the PPI to analyze COVID-19 mitigation policy adoption in Argentina, Brazil, and Mexico from January to December 2020.

3.2 Comparing PPI at the National and Subnational Levels

The PPI is a measure of how stringent COVID-19 policies were at the national and subnational levels in a country on each country-day. In particular, the variable takes into account the extent to which governments closed borders, closed schools, closed businesses, put limits on social gatherings, enacted social distancing policies, established lockdowns, adopted medical isolation procedures, adopted mandatory mask policies, and adopted a state of emergency. Higher values of the index indicate a government adopted more stringent measures for a given day. Also note that more stringent policies in the index, such as lockdowns, are weighted more (Shvetsova et al. 2022).

To begin to compare each government's response to COVID-19 in 2020, I plotted the overall PPIs (dark line), the national PPIs (dashed line), and the overall subnational PPIs (dotted line) in Argentina, Mexico, and Brazil throughout 2020 in Fig. 3.1. In Argentina, the overall stringency of the government response to COVID-19 was much higher than

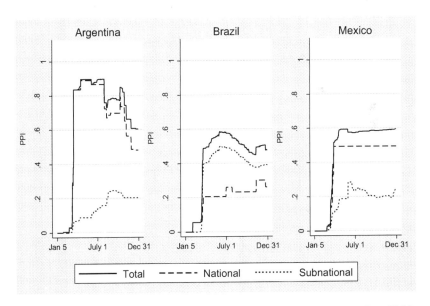

Fig. 3.1 PPI in Argentina, Mexico, and Brazil, January to December 2020. (Source: Shvetsova et al. 2022)

in Brazil and Mexico throughout the year. In addition, in Argentina, the national PPI contributed a great deal to the overall PPI throughout most of the year. In contrast, Brazil and Mexico adopted less stringent measures overall, but the approaches the national and subnational governments adopted in each country differed. In Brazil, the national government had the least stringent response to the pandemic among all three countries, and therefore states took the lead in responding to the pandemic. In Mexico, the national government played a stronger role in responding to the pandemic than in Brazil, but the stringency level was still lower than in Argentina. Mexican states adopted some stringent measures as well, substantively contributing to the country's overall PPI throughout the year.

Hence, based on the PPI, it appears that Argentina's overall and national response to COVID-19 throughout most of 2020 was much more stringent than Brazil's or Mexico's. And while Mexico and Brazil had similar responses, the Brazilian response was state led while the Mexican response was led by both the state and federal governments. In the next three sections I offer several possible explanations as to why all three countries responded differently to the pandemic.

3.3 Argentina's Federal-Led Response to COVID-19

Argentina confirmed its first case of COVID-19 on March 3, 2022. Compared to other countries in the region, Argentina's federal government had the swiftest and most stringent initial response to the virus. The federal government declared a state of emergency, restricted travel, and shut down businesses and schools nationwide. Then, on March 19, it adopted a complete lockdown in the country, which was strictly enforced by security officials. The Federal Police and the National Gendarmerie reported that between March and July, a third of the people in Argentina had been warned to obey the lockdown (Lupien et al. 2021; VanDusky-Allen et al. 2020).

Comparatively higher levels of economic development could partially explain why Argentina was able to adopt more stringent policies nationwide for most of 2020. In addition, having an older, well-established political party in charge at the national level made adopting and implementing stringent policies throughout the country easier. Lastly, since the federal government typically played a strong role in healthcare policymaking in Argentina, it made sense that the federal government played a stronger role than the states did in responding to COVID-19. In what follows, I discuss how economic and political factors influenced Argentina's COVID-19 response.

3.3.1 The Political Economy of Pandemic Policymaking

During the early months of the pandemic, governments in wealthier countries and wealthier regions of a country were in a more comfortable position to adopt more stringent measures. In more developed countries, a larger portion of the population typically works in the service sector. Since many service-sector jobs involve the use of computers, if the government limited economic activity and asked people not to go to work, workers may have still been able to work from home. In addition, given that access to the Internet is more widespread in more developed countries, a significant portion of the labor force would likely be able to still attend work meetings online.

In contrast, governments in poorer countries and poorer regions of a country were less able to adopt stringent measures because of the impact they would have on the most vulnerable citizens in their country. A significant portion of the population likely would not be able to work remotely because they probably had manual labor jobs. If they could not work due to a lockdown, they likely would have lost access to the basic necessities of life. As such, they may have continued to go to work if they could (Bargain and Aminjonov 2021; Lupien et al. 2021).

Entering the pandemic, Argentina was ahead of Brazil and Mexico on a variety of macroeconomic indicators (Table 3.1). Compared to Brazil and Mexico, Argentina had the highest percentage of its population working in services and the lowest in agriculture. Internet usage was also the highest, making remote work more feasible. Argentina also had a higher GDP per capita and a lower poverty rate. Income inequality was also lower (World Bank 2019). Argentina also ranked highest in the Human Development Index (HDI) (United National Development Programme 2019).

Hence, because Argentina was more developed than Brazil and Mexico, the government may have been more willing to adopt stringent measures to mitigate the spread of COVID-19. Since a smaller portion of its population worked in manufacturing and a larger portion worked in services, more workers could have worked from home. The costs to implement a

54   J. VANDUSKY-ALLEN

Table 3.1 Development Indicators Immediately Prior to the Pandemic in Argentina, Brazil, and Mexico

	Argentina	*Brazil*	*Mexico*
GDP per capita	10,056.638	8897.553	9950.45
Poverty (under $5.50/day)	14.4%	19.6%	22.7%
Income inequality	42.9	53.4	45.4
Employment in agriculture	0.06%	9.08%	12.48%
Employment in industry	21.84%	19.99%	25.55%
Employment in services	78.10%	70.94%	61.97%
Internet usage	74.295%	73.912%	70.07%
HDI ranking	48	79	76

Sources: World Bank (2019), United Nations Development Programme (2019)

lockdown in Argentina may have been comparatively lower for a larger portion of the population than in Brazil and Mexico.

It is important to note that, although Argentina had a comparatively higher level of development at this time, entering the pandemic, it was facing an economic decline. It was also facing a sovereign debt crisis and had to default on its debt in May 2020. The strict mitigation measures likely would have strained the Argentine economy even further. Nevertheless, Del Valle et al. (2021) found that Argentina's government has traditionally had a better track record when it comes to alleviating poverty and income inequality compared to other Latin American countries, in part because of long established and generous social welfare programs (Lustig et al. 2014). Therefore, unsurprisingly, at the start of the nationwide lockdown, the government increased benefits to existing social welfare programs. It also quickly created an Emergency Family Income (IFE) program to help families affected the most by the COVID-19 restrictions. So, although the COVID-19 mitigation restrictions would make economic conditions worse in Argentina, the government already had the experience and infrastructure in place to quickly redistribute government resources to families who would be the most impacted by the restrictions (Costabel 2020; Lupien et al. 2021).

3.3.2   *Argentina's Governing Parties*

The history and nature of Argentina's governing parties also likely made it easier for the government to adopt and implement strict mitigation measures (Giraudy et al. 2020). This is despite the fact that Argentina's party system is a series of contradictions. It does have two stable political coalitions on each side of the political spectrum, the left-leaning Frente de Todos and the right-leaning Juntos por el Cambio. The Frente de Todos is led by the Partido Justicialista (PJ), one of the oldest and most well-established parties in Argentina. The PJ has proven to be able to consistently receive a large percentage of votes in presidential elections over time and is capable of winning a plurality of seats in the Chamber of Deputies (Casullo 2021).

Despite Argentina's two stable electoral coalitions and the consistency of PJ over time, Argentina's party system is also highly fragmented. Besides the Unión Cívica Radical (UCR) (which is part of Juntos por el Cambio) and Partido Socialista, most of the other parties in Argentina are relatively young. They are also not able to perform consistently well in national elections. Their ability to attract votes varies significantly from year to year. As such, Argentine elections have been quite volatile throughout the twenty-first century. Additionally, although there appears to be left- and right-leaning parties in Argentina, these parties are not necessarily ideologically consistent over time. This is especially the case when parties form alliances for provincial elections. Parties are willing to form electoral alliances with ideologically different parties if those alliances will help them win votes, and different sets of alliances can form in different provinces and at the national level (Gervasoni 2018).

While Argentina has a somewhat fragmented party system, the president of Argentina, Alberto Fernández, is a member of the oldest and strongest party in the country, the PJ. In contrast, the presidents of Brazil and Mexico are from relatively younger parties (Table 3.2). Since PJ has a long history of governing through crises, this likely helped the president

Table 3.2 Political Indicators Immediately Prior to the Pandemic in Argentina, Brazil, and Mexico

	Argentina	Brazil (previous incumbent)	Mexico
Age of president's party	73 years	25 years	8 years
Percentage of governors that are copartisans with the president	50%	4%	18.8%
Effective number of legislative parties	2.33	16.46	2.12

and the party in developing policies to respond to COVID-19. The party also controls twelve out of the twenty-four governor's positions throughout the country, and three of the other governors are affiliated with Frente de Todos. Since more than half the provinces were either led by PJ governors or governors affiliated with the party, it was likely relatively easier for the federal government to coordinate with provincial governors in adopting and implementing COVID-19 mitigation measures. This is in contrast to Brazil and Mexico, where very few governors were copartisans with the president.

3.3.3 Healthcare Policymaking

The nature of healthcare policymaking in Argentina may have also contributed to the federal government's strong role in responding to COVID-19 (Shvetsova et al. 2021). In Argentina, the government is constitutionally obligated to protect the health of its citizens. In addition, while there is a significant private health insurance sector in Argentina, government-sponsored health care also plays an important role in ensuring all Argentinians have access to health care throughout the country (Rubinstein et al. 2018). Given the government's traditional role in the healthcare system in Argentina, it is not surprising that the federal government played a large role in responding to COVID-19.

It is important to note that in Argentina, the provinces have also played a key role in healthcare provision in Argentina. Had the federal government not adopted stringent COVID-19 policies early on, it is likely the provinces would have adopted them on their own. A handful of provinces did begin to adopt policies right before the federal government placed the country on lockdown. However, as the data in Fig. 3.1 suggest, once the government placed the country on lockdown, the provinces mostly followed the federal government's lead and only slowly adopted policies to supplement the federal government's response.

3.3.4 Summary

Argentina's overall response to COVID-19 was the most stringent among Latin America's federations, and the federal government played a large role in this response. More favorable economic conditions made it easier for the federal government to adopt stringent measures. Having the oldest, most established party in control at the national level and at the state level in half the provinces made it easier for the government to adopt and implement mitigation policies. And given that the federal government typically played a large role in promoting health care in Argentina, it made sense that it continued to play this role during the pandemic.

In the next section I analyze Brazil's response to COVID-19. In contrast to Argentina, Brazil had the least stringent response overall among the federations.

3.4 COVID-19 in Brazil: A State-Led Response

The first confirmed case of COVID-19 in Brazil was on February 25, 2020. President Bolsonaro dismissed the pandemic from the very beginning. He said that most Brazilians would survive the pandemic because they could be dunked in raw sewage and not catch a thing. Even after he tested positive for COVID-19, he played down the severity of the virus, continued to sometimes go maskless in meetings with other people, and claimed COVID-19 was just a little flu (Sulliman 2020). He also criticized officials at the state level for adopting restrictions and even criticized members of the public for following public health guidelines to avoid catching and spreading COVID-19 (Londoño et al. 2020).

Given Bolsonaro's position (Coronavirus Threat to Brazil 2020), it is not surprising that the federal government did not adopt many measures to address the crisis. The federal government adopted a few travel restrictions and a limited work-from-home policy. Otherwise, it adopted few other restrictive measures, such as lockdowns. Instead, the Brazilian states took the lead in mitigating the spread of COVID-19 (VanDusky-Allen et al. 2020). The data from Fig. 3.1 illustrate this dynamic. The overall response to COVID-19 in Brazil was less severe than in Argentina and Mexico throughout all of 2020, and the state-level response was the main contributor to Brazil's overall response.

Although the states took the lead in addressing the pandemic, there was a great deal of variation in how the states responded. It was almost as if each state was its own country, responding to the pandemic in its own way. As such, comparing state-level responses to COVID-19 in Brazil is similar to comparing cross-national responses to the pandemic. Some states adopted few policies; others enacted lockdowns and then adopted phased reopening plans (Shvetsova et al. 2022).

As a result of the federal government's inaction during most of 2020 in combating the pandemic and the variation in state-level responses, Brazil had the least stringent response to COVID-19 among Latin America's

58   J. VANDUSKY-ALLEN

federations. This is surprising given the nature of typical healthcare policy-making in Brazil. The Brazilian constitution guarantees the right to health care, and at least on paper all Brazilians have access to healthcare services (although in practice this varies by region) (Lupien et al. 2021). Hence, we should have expected to observe the Brazilian federal government playing a larger role in addressing COVID-19. To address why Brazil defies expectations, I argue that the level of economic development in Brazil and the structure of Brazil's party system made it more difficult for the federal government to adopt stringent measures and for the country to adopt stringent measures overall. I also argue that at the state level, the partisan affiliation of governors significantly either enhanced or limited the ability of governors to adopt policies.

3.4.1   The Political Economy of Brazil's Response to COVID-19

Economic conditions could partially explain why Brazil's response was comparatively minimal among the federations in Latin America. According to the statistics in Table 3.1, Brazil is less developed than Argentina. It has the lowest GDP per capita and highest income equality among the federations. It also has a higher poverty rate than Argentina and a lower percentage of workers working in services. Given these less favorable economic conditions, COVID-19 mitigation measures likely would have had a stronger negative economic impact on a larger percentage of Brazil's population. Low-income groups would have been the most impacted by strict policies, and this likely would have led them to fall into extreme poverty.

Brazil's size could also explain why the federal government was less likely to adopt blanket mitigation policies that would have applied throughout the country. Brazil is by far the largest of the federations, and the country's overall macroeconomic statistics mask the great deal of variation in development across the Brazilian states. Some states are much worse off than others, and national mitigation policies likely would have worse impacts in some states (United Nations Development Program 2013). As such, adopting a blanket lockdown might have been feasible in some states but not others. Hence, it makes some sense that the federal government allowed the states to lead the response to the pandemic.

It is important to note that, despite not adopting stringent measures at the national level, the federal government did increase social welfare spending to address the negative economic impacts of the pandemic. The Brazilian National Congress increased spending on existing social welfare programs and created temporary social welfare programs to help individuals most affected by the virus (Lupien et al. 2021). These measures made it easier for states to adopt their own mitigation policies.

3.4.2 Party Politics and Brazil's COVID-19 Response

The nature of Brazil's party system also likely limited its ability to adopt stringent policies (Giraudy et al. 2020). Brazil's party system is currently highly fragmented. According to the most recent election, Brazil has 16.46 effective legislative parties (Gallagher 2021). In addition, eleven different parties control the governors' positions at the state level. Given the highly fragmented nature of the party system in Brazil, it might have been difficult for the parties at the level of national and state governments to arrive quickly at a consensus on how to address the spread of COVID-19.

It is also worth noting that Bolsonaro had abandoned his political party in 2019, so he was an independent at the start of the pandemic. In addition, prior to the pandemic, he held extreme views on a variety of political issues and took a contentious approach to politics in Brazil. As such, he had a hard time forming alliances with members of other parties. With limited allies at the state level, he could not rely on preexisting political connections to help him coordinate policies at the state level (Borges and Rennó 2021).

3.4.3 State-Level Responses

Since the federal government in Brazil did not adopt stringent policies, it was up to the Brazilian states to adopt these policies. However, there was a great deal of variation in the state-level responses in Brazil. While states like Amapá tended to adopt more stringent measures, states like Minas Gerais did not. In this section I analyze factors that might have impacted the stringency of policies at the state level in Brazil. I expect that case rates would have positively impacted the stringency of measures in Brazil at the state level. As case rates increased, states should have adopted more stringent measures. Second, I expect poverty rates to have had a negative impact on the stringency of measures. As poverty increased, the stringency of measures should have decreased. I also controlled for the governor's partisan affiliation. Different parties may have adopted different policies due to ideological and/or strategic reasons.

To analyze the impact of case rates, poverty rates, and partisan politics on the stringency of state-level COVID-19 policies, I use data from the PPI dataset at the state level in Brazil from March 19 to December 31, 2020. The unit of analysis is the state-day. Since the dataset is organized as a cross-sectional time series and PPI at the state level on any given day is correlated with the state's previous day's PPI, I ran a series of generalized estimating equations (GEEs) assuming one-day autocorrelated errors.

The first independent variable in the analysis was *cases per capita* (Brazil Ministry of Health 2022). This variable should have a positive impact on PPI. The second independent variable was *poverty*. I used data from the Instituto de Pesquisa Econômica Aplicada (2014) in Brazil to measure poverty rates in a state. This variable should have a negative impact on PPI. I also included a series of dummy variables that captured which party a governor belonged to. The reference and excluded category was Progressistas, a center-right-wing party.

Table 3.3 presents the model's results, which suggest that *cases per capita* and *poverty* rates do not impact the stringency of mitigation measures at the state level in the way that I expect. The coefficients for several of the parties are significant, however. Governors from the social-democratic Partido Democrático Trabalhista (PDT) adopted more stringent measures than governors from right-leaning Progressistas. Governors from the center-left-leaning Partido dos Trabalhadores (PT), the center-right Movimento Democrático Brasileiro (MDB), the center-right Partido da Social Democracia Brasileira (PSDB), the center-right Partido Novo (NOVO), and the far right Partido Social Liberal (PSL) adopted less stringent measures.

These results can in part explain why states like Amapá adopted more stringent measures than average. The governor of Amapá, Waldez Góes, was a member of the left-leaning PDT, which adopted more stringent measures according to the regression analysis performed. Governor Góes's public statements about the pandemic indicated that he believed the restrictions would help control the spread of COVID-19 and save lives (Globo 2020). In contrast, the results from the analysis can also explain why states like Minas Gerais adopted less stringent measures. The governor of Minas Gerais, Romeu Zema, was a member of the right-leaning NOVO, which adopted less stringent measures according to the regression analysis. Governor Zema's statements about the pandemic indicated that he thought the government should take a limited role in fighting the pandemic despite the death toll. In interviews, he criticized mayors for

Table 3.3 Brazilian State-Level COVID-19 Policies (Robust Standard Errors in Parentheses)

	Model 1
Cases per Capita	-0.582
	(1.456)
Poverty	0.002
	(0.001)
PDT	0.153**
	(0.060)
UNIÃO	-0.027
	(0.044)
PT	-0.089*
	(0.042)
MDB	-0.141**
	(0.049)
PSB	-0.051
	(0.049)
PSDB	-0.110**
	(0.045)
NOVO	-0.178**
	(0.063)
PSC	-0.079
	(0.061)
Republican	0.034
	(0.065)
PSL	-0.230***
	(0.060)
Constant	0.427***
	(0.046)
N	7618
Prob > chi²	0.0000

$*p < 0.05; **p < 0.01; ***p < 0.001$

adopting stringent policies, arguing that it was not a problem for COVID-19 to spread a little (Leite 2020). In other interviews he argued that, despite Brazil's limited overall response to COVID-19 and the high number of deaths, he thought the government responded appropriately to the pandemic (Ronan 2020).

Although case rates and poverty rates did not impact state-level responses, it is clear from the results that party politics played a significant role in state-level responses. Borges and Rennó (2021) observed a similar pattern in Brazil throughout the pandemic. They argued that, since Bolsonaro was such a polarizing figure in Brazilian politics, his opponents felt it was important to take a stance on the pandemic that contrasted with his. Since the federal government played a limited role in addressing the pandemic, governors from opposition parties coordinated their state-level responses and adopted their own policies. Of course, not all opposition governors adopted the most stringent policies. However, the incentives did exist for them at the very least to adopt more stringent policies than the federal government did.

3.4.4 Summary

Brazil's response to COVID-19 was unusual. Typically, the Brazilian federal government would play a large role in responding to a pandemic. Yet it did not. The federal government played a small role in addressing COVID-19, and the states played a larger role, and the overall response to COVID-19 in Brazil was limited. I contend that challenges to development throughout Brazil made it harder for the federal government to adopt national policies to mitigate the spread of COVID-19. Those policies would have drastic negative economic impacts on the poorest states in Brazil. Additionally, since the federal government was led by a young populist who denied the severity of the pandemic threat, it was less willing to adopt stringent measures. A fragmented party system also made it harder for the federal government to coordinate with the states on pandemic policymaking since none of the governors were copartisans with the president.

Although the federal government did not adopt stringent policies to combat COVID-19, some of the states did. In this section I also examined factors that influenced these state-led responses. I found that at the state level, case and poverty rates did not impact the stringency of policies that governors adopted. Instead, partisanship influenced the stringency of measures. Governors from more right-leaning parties typically adopted less stringent policies than more centrist parties. In the next section, I analyze the combined federal-state response to COVID-19 in Mexico.

3.5 The Combined Federal-State Response to COVID-19 in Mexico

On February 28, 2020, the Mexican government confirmed the country's first COVID-19 case. In response, both the federal and state governments adopted a series of mitigation measures to manage the initial spread of

COVID-19 throughout Mexico. The federal government declared a state of emergency, closed nonessential businesses and entertainment venues, closed schools, placed restrictions on social gatherings, adopted work from home policies, and partially closed the borders. While the states overall played a smaller role in responding to COVID-19, many governors also made emergency declarations, closed businesses and entertainment venues, placed restrictions on social gatherings, and limited travel between states. Some states even adopted more stringent measures than the federal government did, such as adopting mask mandates early on (VanDusky-Allen et al. 2020).

After the pandemic onset period (from June 1, 2020), the federal government led a reopening plan for the country based on a traffic-light system. During this period, the federal government assessed the COVID-19 risk for each state every week based on a variety of health indicators such as state-level incidence rates, mortality rates, hospitalization rates, and number of beds with ventilators occupied in the last fourteen days. Based on these data, the federal government classified states as red (the most at risk), orange, yellow, and green (the least at risk) and suggested specific policies for states to adopt to address COVID-19 within their states. The states did not have to adopt these policies. State governments adopted stricter policies or less strict policies (Secretaría de Salud 2020).[1]

Although throughout most of 2020 both federal and state governments in Mexico adopted measures to address COVID-19, the overall total stringency of measures in Mexico was lower than in Argentina and comparable to Brazil's response. I argue that the nature of Mexico's labor force, the level of economic development in Mexico, and the structure of Mexico's ruling parties made it more difficult for the government to adopt stringent measures.

In addition to analyzing the overall stringency of COVID-19 mitigation measures in Mexico, I also analyze how federalism and healthcare policymaking influenced the federal and state governments' roles in responding to COVID-19. With respect to the pandemic onset period, I argue that the federal government in Mexico likely played a stronger role

---

[1] Note that this made coding Mexico a bit difficult for this period as the federal government supported stringent measures for some states and not others, and states were allowed to ignore the advice of the federal government. As such, while the overall stringency of the PPI for Mexico remains high for this time, as the federal government endorsed stringent policies, the complex interplay between federal and state policymaking likely meant that in practice overall stringency was lower than the PPI can capture.

64   J. VANDUSKY-ALLEN

in responding to COVID-19 than the states did because the federal government is institutionally accountable for healthcare provision, and it typically plays a large role in healthcare financing. In addition, at the state level, I also argue that economic conditions, health conditions, and political conditions within each individual state also influenced the extent to which individual states adopted COVID-19 mitigation measures.

3.5.1   *The Political Economy of Mexico's Response to COVID-19*

Compared to Argentina, Mexico had a less stringent response to COVID-19. Economic conditions could partially explain this variation. Mexico lags behind Argentina on a variety of economic indicators (Table 3.1). It has a lower GDP per capita, higher income inequality, a higher percentage of its population living in poverty, and a lower human development index. COVID-19 mitigation measures likely would have had a stronger negative economic impact on a larger percentage of the population in Mexico. Furthermore, it is notable that a much larger percentage of Mexico's workforce works in the industrial sector. The shutdowns had a significant negative impact on manufacturing production in Mexico, which directly impacted a large portion of the labor force. Additionally, Mexico has the lowest portion of its labor force working in services and the lowest portion of its population that used the Internet. As such, remote work is less of a possibility for a large portion of the population.

Given the nature of Mexico's labor force, it is not surprising that the national government was initially hesitant to adopt lockdowns, especially in the manufacturing sector. Even after it shut down factories, the government was reluctant to keep them closed. Hence, even before the federal government lifted restrictive measures in June, it began a very limited targeted reopening of factories in May 2020 (Zissis 2020). It was clear that the economic cost of keeping factories closed outweighed the health benefits for the federal government.

It is also important to note that the federal government was one of the least reluctant governments in Latin America to address the economic effects of the pandemic. It was not until April that the president proposed his modest plan to combat the negative economic impacts. However, unlike Brazil and Argentina, the Mexican government did not plan to create a specific COVID-19 cash transfer program to help those most effected by COVID-19. Instead, it only increased funds for existing social welfare programs. In addition, the total cost of the plan as a percentage of GDP was well below most other countries' economic recovery plans. As such, while the federal government was willing to adopt some stringent policies to address the pandemic, it was far less likely to support the economic side effects of those policies. This may be why it was reluctant to adopt even more stringent policies, as it did not want to address the costs of those policies (Lupien et al. 2021).

3.5.2 Party Politics and Mexico's COVID-19 Response

Another factor that likely limited Mexico's national response was party politics (Giraudy et al. 2020). Although Mexico has a more institutionalized party system than Argentina (Greene and Sánchez-Talanquer 2018); it has several older, well-established parties that typically compete for power (PRI, PAN, and PRD), and at the time of the pandemic, a very young left-leaning populist party, MORENA, was in control of the presidency, the Chamber of Deputies, and the Senate. Hence, throughout the pandemic, the youngest, least established, and least experienced party in Mexico controlled the federal government. The lack of experience with leading the policymaking process, especially during a crisis, likely hindered MORENA's ability to offer a strong response to the pandemic.

It is also noteworthy that MORENA only controlled six out of the thirty-two states in Mexico. Cross-partisan divisions may have limited MORENA's ability to enact a strong nationwide response to the pandemic as governors had little experience coordinating with MORENA during the policymaking process. Furthermore, most of the states were governed by the older, more-established parties in Mexico. This could in part explain why the federal government relied on states to lead the COVID-19 effort, especially after June 1, 2020. These parties were more likely to have the experience to adopt and implement the appropriate measures to address the pandemic.

MORENA's populist leanings also likely influenced its limited response to COVID-19. Analyzing the national government's response to the pandemic, Renteria and Arellano-Gault (2021) found that key members of the government held negative beliefs about expert scientific opinion and were uninterested in seeking out more information to help respond to the pandemic. This slowed down the federal government's response to the pandemic and limited its willingness to adopt stringent measures.

3.5.3   Healthcare Policymaking

While the overall response to COVID-19 in Mexico was less stringent than in Argentina, in both countries the federal government played a stronger role in responding to the pandemic than the states did during the pandemic onset period. As in Argentina, the nature of healthcare policymaking in Mexico may have also contributed to the federal government's strong role in responding to COVID-19 (Shvetsova et al. 2021). The Mexican government is constitutionally obligated to protect the health of its citizens, and in Mexico, the federal government has traditionally played a large role in financing health care. Hence, it is not surprising that the federal government played a large role in responding to COVID-19 early on. Nonetheless, after June 1, the states began to play a bigger role in responding to the pandemic. This contradicts my expectations that the federal government would have continued to take the lead in responding to the pandemic. However, given MORENA's populist leanings and aversion to to expert opinion, it is not surprising that the federal government would want to delegate to the states responsibility for addressing the pandemic in their own way. In addition, once again, it not surprising that the more traditional, mainstream parties in Mexico at the state level wanted to play a larger role in responding to the pandemic as they had more experience in policymaking during crises.

3.5.4   State-Level Responses

Given that states also played a role in responding to COVID-19 in Mexico, it is important to understand what influenced the extent to which states adopted COVID-19 policies. Hence, in this section, I analyze factors that influenced state-level responses.

First, using the PPI measure, I qualitatively compared each state's response during the onset phase of the pandemic (between February 2 and June 1, 2020) and then compared them during the traffic-light phase after June 1, 2020. During the onset phase there was a great deal of variation within each state's initial response. Some states adopted very few policies, while others adopted policies that were nearly as restrictive as the federal government's. I observe a similar pattern during the traffic-light period of the pandemic after June 1. There was a great deal of variation in state governments' responses to COVID-19, with some states adopting stringent measures and others adopting very few measures.

What can account for the variation in state-level responses to COVID-19 throughout 2020? Given that the federal and state governments were both likely taking into account case rates when determining which policies to adopt, we would expect daily case rates per capita in a country to have a positive effect on the stringency of mitigation measures. As the number of cases increased, state governments should have been more likely to increase restrictions on citizens' behavior in order to mitigate the spread of COVID-19 within their states.

Poverty rates within a state also likely influenced state governments' willingness to adopt strict mitigation measures. If governments in poorer regions had adopted stringent policies, that could have pushed the most vulnerable populations in their regions into extreme poverty. They likely would not have been able to fully enforce the policies as people might have continued to work to avoid starvation or homelessness (Bargain and Aminjonov 2021). As such, as poverty rates increased, state officials were probably less likely to adopt measures that restricted behavior.

The nature of party politics in Mexico could also have affected which policies state governments adopted. Parties may have taken different approaches to addressing pandemic. Ideological considerations could have driven the parties' perspectives on the government's role in managing the spread of COVID-19. Strategic political considerations could also have influenced their responses.

To analyze the impact of case rates, poverty rates, and partisan politics on the stringency of state-level COVID-19 policies, I use data from the PPI dataset at the state level in Mexico from March 26 to December 31, 2020. The unit of analysis is the state-day. Since the dataset is organized as a cross-sectional time series and PPI at the state level on any given day is correlated with the state's previous day's PPI, I ran a series of GEEs assuming one-day autocorrelated errors.

The first independent variable in the analysis was *cases per capita*. I used data from the Health Secretary of the Mexican government (2022) to measure a state's COVID-19 case rate per capita on a given day. This variable should have a positive impact on PPI. The second independent variable was *poverty*. I used data from the OECD (2015) to measure poverty rates in a state. This variable should have a negative impact on PPI. I also included a series of dummy variables that captured which party a governor belonged to. The reference and excluded category was MORENA.

I present the results of the model in Table 3.4. The coefficient for *cases per capita* was positive and significant at the 0.01 level. As expected, as the

68   J. VANDUSKY-ALLEN

Table 3.4 Mexican State-Level COVID-19 Policies (Robust Standard Errors in Parentheses)

	Model 2
Cases per capita	16.343**
	(6.667)
Poverty	-0.002*
	(0.001)
PAN	-0.020
	(0.042)
PRI	-0.036
	(0.038)
MC	0.147*
	(0.083)
PRD	0.015
	(0.061)
PV	-0.013
	(0.081)
Independent	-0.105
	(0.088)
Constant	0.275
	(0.066)
N	9920
Prob > chi^2	0.0317

$*p < 0.05; **p < 0.01; ***p < 0.001$

number of cases increased, mitigation policies increased. The coefficient for *poverty* was negative and significant at the 0.05 level. As poverty increased in a state, mitigation measures decreased. As for the party dummy variables, only the coefficient for the MC was significant, indicating that, for the most part, governor's partisanship did not impact the stringency of COVID-19 policies compared to governors from MORENA, the president's party.

The results of the regression analysis for Mexico are in stark contrast to the results for Brazil. While *cases per capita* and *poverty* had a significant impact on the extent to which Mexican governors adopted mitigation policies, they did not in Brazil. And yet in Brazil, partisan considerations played a large role in state-level responses, but not in Mexico. What explains these differences? Perhaps Mexico's prior experience with H1N1 could in part explain why governors in Mexico took a more policy-centric and less partisan approach to adopting COVID-19 mitigation policies.

In retrospect, the federal and state governments in Mexico did not handle H1N1 well. While in early 2009 the Mexican government noticed an increase in pneumonia cases in the country, they assumed it was just the flu. It was not until April 11 that they detected H1N1. It was not until ten days later that they fully informed the population of the situation. Within that time period, the virus spread, and several people died as a result of misdiagnosis. State and local governments finally began to adopt measures on April 23. That is when the government of Mexico City and some state governments began to shut down schools and businesses. Public officials also began to encourage widespread mask wearing and use of hand sanitizer as a preventive measure (Cavalcanti 2021).

The former secretary of health during H1N1 in Mexico noted that after H1N1, the Mexican government made a series of changes to healthcare policymaking. Of note, they improved risk communication procedures to help encourage the population to voluntarily comply with mitigation measures. They also strengthened the national network of public health laboratories and the antiviral drug distribution system (Cavalcanti 2021).

For their part, it does appear that the Mexican state governments did learn some lessons from H1N1 and applied some of those lessons to handling COVID-19. The Mexican state governments took a less partisan approach to addressing the pandemic. Instead, they took a more policy-centric approach to adopting mitigation measures. When cases increased, they increased the stringency of the measures in an effort to control the spread of COVID-19. But they also took into account the economic impact these measures would have and adopted less stringent measures if the economic impact would be felt too strongly within a state. Of course, this is not to say that collectively the measures effectively controlled the spread of COVID-19. The limited coordination between the federal and state governments made it harder for the country as a whole to address the pandemic. This could in part explain why, throughout the pandemic, Mexico had one of the worst COVID-19 case and death rates in the world (Natal 2021).

3.6 Conclusion

At the start of the COVID-19 pandemic, health officials promoted a series of measures to combat the spread of COVID-19 throughout the world. But governments' willingness to adopt these measures varied. Even if political institutions, like federalism, charged different levels of government with safeguarding the public's health, if the officials that occupied those positions were unwilling to take the appropriate measures to fight the pandemic, then the government was less likely to adopt stringent mitigation policies. This limited public health officials' and healthcare professionals' ability to help check the spread of COVID-19. Hence, to prepare for future pandemics, it is important to identify factors that make government officials more or less likely to address a global public health crisis.

In this chapter I identified three factors that could affect whether a government will adopt mitigation measures during a pandemic: economic development, the nature of political parties and party systems, and the role of the government in the healthcare system. With respect to development, scholars have long acknowledged that development has a positive impact on public health. The COVID-19 pandemic has shown that economic development is also essential during a public health crisis because it will impact whether a government can respond to the crisis. In the face of inequality and poverty, governments may not be able to adopt strict lockdowns to mitigate the spread of a virus. Hence, to prepare for future crises, governments and development-focused organizations should develop ways to address the short-term negative economic impacts of restrictive healthcare policies.

With respect to the role of governments in healthcare provision, governments throughout the world should reflect back on their experiences handling the pandemic and reevaluate how their governments address healthcare crises. They should consider what role the government should play, how to prevent that role from being politicized, and how to prepare future leaders to address healthcare crises. This is especially the case in federations where two levels of government could potentially address a crisis. Leaders should consider how national and subnational governments could coordinate their efforts, especially when leaders come from different partisan backgrounds.

As for the nature of the party system and parties themselves, fragmented, less institutionalized party systems make it harder for governments to respond to a health crisis, as does the rise of populist parties. However, these phenomena are often just a natural part of the democratic process. As such, it is unlikely that leaders can prevent these conditions from evolving in their country. Instead, when leaders formulate plans to respond to a future public health crisis, they should consider what might happen under various partisan conditions and develop approaches to addressing the impacts these conditions could have on a given response to the public health crisis.

REFERENCES

Bargain O, Aminjonov U (2021) Poverty and COVID-19 in Africa and Latin America. World Dev 142: 105422.

Borges A, Rennó L (2021) Brazilian Response to COVID-19: Polarization and Conflict. In: Fernandez M, Machado C (eds) COVID-19's political challenges in Latin America. Springer, Cham, p 9–22.

Brazil Ministry of Health (2022) COVID-19 Statistics. https://covid.saude.gov.br/.

Cavalcanti B (2021) Mexico in the Face of COVID-19: In-Between Actions and Inefficiency. In: Fernandez M, Machado C (eds) COVID-19's political challenges in Latin America. Springer, Cham, p 23–33.

Casullo ME (2021) Why Argentina's Politics Are Surprisingly Stable. Americas Quarterly. https://www.americasquarterly.org/article/why-argentinas-politics-are-surprisingly-stable/.

Coronavirus Threat to Brazil (2020). The New York Times, April 1. https://www.nytimes.com/2020/04/01/world/americas/brazil-bolsonaro-coronavirus.html.

Costabel M (2020) Argentina's Economy Crumbles as Buenos Aires Lockdown Continues. Foreign Policy. https://foreignpolicy.com/2020/08/27/argentina-economy-crumbles-buenos-aires-lockdown-continues/.

Del Valle JCL, López CB, Campabadal J et al (2021) Fiscal Policy, Income Redistribution and Poverty Reduction in Argentina. No. 111. Tulane University, Department of Economics, 2021.

Gallagher M (2021) Election indices dataset. http://www.tcd.ie/Political_Science/people/michael_gallagher/ElSystems/index.php.

Gervasoni C (2018) Argentina's declining party system: Fragmentation, denationalization, factionalization, personalization, and increasing fluidity. In: Mainwaring S (ed) Party Systems in Latin America: Institutionalization, Decay, and Collapse. Cambridge University Press, Cambridge, p 255–290.

Giraudy A, Niedzwiecki S, Pribble J (2020) How Political Science Explains Countries' Reactions to COVID-19. Americas Quarterly. https://www.americasquarterly.org/article/how-political-science-explains-countries-reactions-to-covid-19/.

Globo (2020) Coronavírus: governo decide suspender atividades no Amapá para limitar circulação de pessoas. Globo. https://g1.globo.com/ap/amapa/noticia/2020/03/19/coronavirus-governo-do-amapa-decide-suspender-atividades-para-limitar-circulacao-de-pessoas.ghtml.

Greene KF, Sánchez-Talanquer M (2018) Authoritarian Legacies and Party System Stability in Mexico. In: Mainwaring S (ed) Party Systems in Latin America: Institutionalization, Decay, and Collapse. Cambridge University Press, Cambridge, p 201–226.

Health Secretary, Mexican Government (2022) Datos, COVID-19. https://datos.covid-19.conacyt.mx/#DownZCSV.

Instituto de Pesquisa Econômica Aplicada (2014) ipeadata, número de domicílios pobres. http://www.ipeadata.gov.br/Default.aspx.

Leite D (2020) Zema critica prefeitos e diz que coronavírus tem que 'viajar um pouco.' UOL, November 4. https://noticias.uol.com.br/politica/ultimas-noticias/2020/04/11/zema-critica-prefeitos-e-diz-que-coronavirus-tem-que-viajar-um-pouco.htm.

Londoño E, Andreoni M, Casado L (2020) Bolsonaro, Isolated and Defiant, Dismisses.

Lupien P, Rincón A, Carrera F et al (2021) Early COVID-19 Policy Responses in Latin America: A Comparative Analysis of Social Protection and Health Policy. Can J Lat Am 46(2): 297–317.

Lustig N, Pessino C, Scott J (2014) The impact of taxes and social spending on inequality and poverty in Argentina, Bolivia, Brazil, Mexico, Peru, and Uruguay: Introduction to the special issue. Public Finance Rev 42(3): 287–303.

Natal A (2021) For the Sake of All, the Poor First: COVID-19, Mañaneras, and the Popularity of the Mexican President. In: Fernandez M, Machado C (eds) COVID-19' political challenges in Latin America. Springer, Cham, p 163–181.

Organization for Economic Cooperation and Development (OECD) (2015) Measuring Well-Being in Mexican States. https://www.oecd.org/cfe/region-aldevelopment/Mexican-States-Highlights-English.pdf.

Renteria C, Arellano-Gault D (2021) How does a populist government interpret and face a health crisis? Evidence from the Mexican populist response to COVID-19. Revista de Administração Pública 55: 180–196.

Ronan G (2020) "O Brasil não fez um trabalho tão ruim", diz Zema sobre pandemia da COVID-19. Estado de Minas, August 3. https://www.em.com.br/app/noticia/gerais/2020/08/03/interna_gerais,1172708/nao-fez-um-trabalho-tao-ruim-diz-zema-sobre-bolsonaro-na-pandemia.shtml.

Rubinstein A, Zerbino MC, Cejas C et al (2018) Making universal health care effective in Argentina: a blueprint for reform. HS&R 4(3): 203–213.

Secretaría de Salud (2020) Lineamiento para la estimación de riesgos del semáforo por regions COVID-19. August 14, 2020. https://coronavirus.gob.mx/wp-content/uploads/2020/10/SemaforoCOVID_Metodo.pdf.

Shvetsova O, VanDusky-Allen J, Zhirnov A et al (2021) Federal Institutions and Strategic Policy Responses to COVID-19 Pandemic. Front Polit Sci 3: 66.

Shvetsova O, Zhirnov A, Adeel AB et al (2022) Protective Policy Index (PPI) global dataset of institutional origins and relative stringency of COVID-19 mitigation policies. Sci Data 9(1): 1–10.

Sulliman A (2020) Bolsonaro dismissed the coronavirus. His positive test highlights Brazil's deadly outbreak. NBC News, July 8. https://www.nbcnews.

com/news/world/bolsonaro-dismissed-coronavirus-his-positive-test-highlights-brazil-s-deadly-n1233135.

The World Bank (2019) World Development Indicators. Washington, D.C.: The World Bank. https://data.worldbank.org/.

United Nations Development Program (2013) O índice de desenvolvimento humano municipal Brasileiro. https://www.ipea.gov.br/portal/images/stories/PDFs/130729_AtlasPNUD_2013.pdf.

United Nations Development Programme (2019) Human Development Report 2019. New York: New York.

VanDusky-Allen J, Shvetsova S, Zhirnov A (2020) COVID-19 Policy Response in Argentina, Brazil, and Mexico: Three Different National-Subnational Approaches. The Duck of Minerva. https://www.duckofminerva.com/2020/07/covid-19-policy-response-in-argentina-brazil-and-mexico-three-different-national-subnational-approaches.html.

Zissis C (2020) Mexico Kick-starts Its Reopening Plan. Americas Society/ Council of the Americas. https://www.as-coa.org/articles/mexico-kick-starts-its-reopening-plan.

CHAPTER 4

COVID-19 Response in India, Pakistan, and Bangladesh: Shared History, Different Processes

Abdul Basit Adeel and Andrei Zhirnov

4.1 Introduction

Whether and how the process of politics matters are among the core questions in social science. In times of crises—such as the COVID-19 pandemic—when politicians are under time pressure to make decisions that carry visible consequences for citizens' health, these questions acquire additional normative value. At such times, disagreements over what is to be done, how, and by whom can and often do take a heavy toll on the public. Especially in federations where national and regional leaders answer to different constituencies, which sometimes generates diagonal incentives and free-riding problems as leaders scramble to opt for the least costly

---

A. B. Adeel
The Pennsylvania State University, State College, PA, USA
e-mail: axa6372@psu.edu

A. Zhirnov (✉)
University of Exeter, Exeter, UK
e-mail: A.Zhirnov@exeter.ac.uk

© The Author(s), under exclusive license to Springer Nature Switzerland AG 2023
O. Shvetsova (ed.), *Government Responses to the COVID-19 Pandemic*, https://doi.org/10.1007/978-3-031-30844-4_4

75

policy scenarios in times of crisis (Wibbels 2005), such political conflict could stifle an efficient public health reaction (Benton 2020; Lecours et al. 2021). Hence, understanding whether and how such conflict matters and how it can be avoided is a critical institutional design question.

We set out to address these questions by investigating how India, Pakistan, and Bangladesh—three South Asian nations—responded to the COVID-19 pandemic. These countries' similarities are many. They share a subcontinent, have a history of being under the same colonial rule, and face similar sanitary, healthcare, and socioeconomic challenges. Similarly high levels of poverty mean that politicians in all three countries face similar trade-offs between securing public health and securing economic livelihoods. All three countries also have similar formal frameworks for dealing with epidemic diseases: they all enjoy a combination of a public health rules document—in the case of India and Pakistan, it was inherited from the British Raj—and the relevant provisions of disaster management regulations.

These similarities enable us to observe differences in the politics of the epidemic response in comparable structural contexts and speculate about the causes of such differences. We trace the similarities and differences in the trajectories of the public health responses in these countries and examine the prevailing mechanisms of interactions among the federal and subnational governments regarding those policies. We also scrutinize the role of institutional frameworks in the formulation of responses to the pandemic, identify the key actors in the pandemic response, and pinpoint the junctions at which the policy trajectories started diverging.

We find that the governments in these countries used similar policy toolkits, but the political interactions and the resulting trajectories of their responses ended up being quite dissimilar. They initially imposed lockdowns in the onset phase, i.e., in the latter half of March, but ended up replacing lockdowns with localized, cluster-containment strategies in the May to June period, when the infections were still on the rise. Despite the apparent similarities in such imposed policies, we observe notable differences in the politics of COVID-19 responses among these countries. These include the contrasting modes of interactions between federal and subnational governments in India and Pakistan, which, despite having similar formal frameworks for public health response, exhibited different patterns of conflict and cooperation. The policymaking process in Pakistan produced an open political conflict between the federal and provincial governments, which escalated to the involvement of both the military and the Supreme Court in the process. Contrary to the cases of India and

Pakistan, the policymaking in Bangladesh involved significant delegation to health authorities.

We then attempt to situate these responses in a broader historical context to explain this apparent variation. We suspect that the variation is partly due to the differential development of public health frameworks and partly due to the variation in the political context in which they operate. We present an overview of the development of epidemic response systems and identify critical events in the transformation of those systems, such as the adoption of the Epidemic Diseases Act of 1897 and the creation of disaster management frameworks in these countries. We argue that the British Raj neither created a broad-access public healthcare system nor a framework for a community-wide epidemic response coupled with the former. It by and large avoided the conflict that would have been involved in wider public health measures by limiting them to ports and urban areas. At the time, this contributed to a situation where many infectious diseases became endemic in the Indian subcontinent. The novelty and limited success of attempts to update such frameworks in modern Bangladesh, India, and Pakistan are partially responsible for the early abandonment of community-wide mitigation measures and the involvement of unexpected actors and the influence of political (rather than healthcare) factors in the process of formulating such responses, including ideology and the existing practices of intergovernmental interactions. The COVID-19 pandemic presents an opportunity (a potential critical juncture) for institutional development.

The rest of the chapter is organized as follows. We start by presenting an analytical framework to trace the trajectory of public health interventions by the respective governments and then describe the timeline of the COVID-19 response in the three countries, highlighting the similarities and differences in the approaches taken to addressing the pandemic. This is followed by an examination of the differences in the institutional frameworks set up for the epidemic response and the actual roles played by major actors in the formulation of COVID-19 measures. Finally, we discuss the legacy of the British Raj and its role in the epidemic response in 2020 within a historical institutionalism framework and predict further institutional developments in the public health arena by treating the COVID-19 pandemic as a critical juncture that could break the institutional path dependence in these countries. We conclude by reiterating that variation in these cases is a result of the absence of a comprehensive pandemic management framework.

4.2 Two Dimensions of Public Health Response

We approach the comparison of the COVID-19 responses in India, Pakistan, and Bangladesh using two analytical dimensions. The first dimension is the overall trajectory of the public health intervention by government. Table 4.1 shows a classification of interventions that a government or government agency can adopt in response to an infectious disease outbreak. Those may be medical and nonmedical and affect only select individuals or areas or the community at large.

The only types of response we see outside of an epidemic are targeted medical actions: patients with symptoms contact a medical facility and are tested and receive treatment if diagnosed and a treatment is available. During outbreaks, governments resort to other types of action, in isolation and in combination with one another. They can implement targeted restrictions on the movements of suspected or likely carriers of the infection or, if such individuals cannot be positively identified, apply forms of cluster containment. Governments can implement broad-based vaccination campaigns if vaccines are available and use lockdowns, restrictions on interpersonal interactions, closures of public venues, and other measures indiscriminately applied to large segments of the community.

These actions vary, among other things, in terms of feasibility (e.g., one cannot administer vaccines against virus X if such vaccines have not been invented), implementation costs and effectiveness, and the disruption caused to routines. Indiscriminate nonmedical interventions incur the highest costs to the routines of the public and are generally avoided by democratic governments (Shvetsova et al. 2021). During the COVID-19 pandemic, governments around the world had to resort to these indiscriminate nonmedical measures; however, they reached and

Table 4.1 Feasible types of action in response to an infectious disease outbreak

	Medical	Nonmedical
Targeted	Testing of symptomatic patients Treatment …	Quarantine Cluster containment …
Indiscriminate	Mass vaccination Mass testing …	Stay-at-home orders Curfews Closures of public venues …

transitioned from the stage at which they applied them in different manners. The packages of such measures varied in their content and paths of implementation.

The second dimension of our analysis are the patterns of interactions among governments in the formulation of COVID-19 policy responses. Epidemic response is a complex task requiring coordination across multiple actors who can, in principle, take actions to protect public health (Adeel et al. 2020; Lecours et al. 2021; Schnabel and Hegele 2021; Shvetsova et al. 2021). Such an ability to act can, in principle, result in all governments acting and all waiting simultaneously for others to take the first step. It can also involve failures to arrive at coordinated procurement, regulation, and information policies. We will look at which governments within the government participated in the pandemic response and how intergovernmental interactions in connection with the pandemic response were organized. Later in the chapter, we also place these interactions in a historical context to inform readers about the trajectory of institutional development in the public health arena in these countries.

4.3 Setting the Stage

Before discussing the trajectory of government responses to the COVID-19 pandemic in India, Pakistan, and Bangladesh (and the historical trajectories leading to them), it is important to first set the stage and introduce the main actors and basic legal documents governing the epidemic response. This will provide some context for the discussion of the cases. We will see who could, in principle, contribute to the making of public health policies and the formal powers and responsibilities they had in this area.

Rarely offering guidance on the specific actions to be taken, public health frameworks can be viewed as power-sharing blueprints, which are supposed to define the options available to politicians, shape the expectations of political actors and the public alike, facilitate coordination among the relevant policymakers, and preempt their conflict. These documents were not always followed to the letter; some actors took proactive steps in areas outside of their direct purview, while others took a laid-back approach despite being in charge, with similar deviations observable in the interactions among them. Nevertheless, the formal rules offer some insight about how the decisions about the epidemic response were made.

Incidentally, our description of institutional and public health frameworks will also serve to emphasize the similarity between the formal structures of government and epidemic response in India and Pakistan and the similarities in the limited reach of the public healthcare systems in the three cases under consideration.

4.3.1 Political System

India and Pakistan are federations. As of early 2020, India comprised twenty-eight states and eight union territories. Both federal and state governments are parliamentary, with a cabinet of ministers—the executive branch—selected by and directly accountable to the legislature. The national politics is dominated by two alliances built around the right-wing Bharatiya Janata Party (BJP) and the Indian National Congress (INC), each relying on the support of regional parties in the national legislature. As of early 2020, the national government was led by Narendra Modi, the leader of BJP and the National Democratic Alliance.

Pakistan is also a federation but is composed of fewer subnational units: four provinces and three territories with special status and just recently, in 2010, underwent major constitutional reform, increasing the autonomy of provinces and reducing the powers of the president, making it a parliamentary republic. National politics is dominated by three national parties: Pakistan Muslim League (Nawaz), Pakistan Tehreek-e-Insaf (PTI), and Pakistan Peoples Party (PPP), national parties with regional strongholds. As of early 2020, the government was led by Imran Khan of PTI. This government would be forced to resign in April 2022.

Unlike India and Pakistan, Bangladesh was created as a unitary republic. Like India and Pakistan, its government is parliamentary, with the executive branch selected by and accountable to the national legislature. The politics of Bangladesh is dominated by the Awami League, which since 2018 has controlled over 80% of seats in the national assembly. As of early 2020, the government has been led by Sheikh Hasina Wazed. Note also that in early 2020, all three countries were led by political leaders with strong personal styles of government, which, in different ways, were imprinted on the way events unfolded.

4.3.2 Healthcare System Administration

None of the three countries has a sufficiently broadly access public healthcare system. There are about 8 hospital beds and 6.4 medical doctors per 10,000 population in Bangladesh, 5.3 hospital beds and 7.3 medical doctors per 10,000 population in India, and 6.3 hospital beds and 11 medical doctors per 10,000 in Pakistan (World Health Organization, n.d.-b). For comparison, the same statistics for the UK are 25 beds and 29 doctors. The private sector bears a large share of healthcare expenses: according to the World Health Organization (WHO) (n.d.-a), in 2019 in Bangladesh, 73% of current healthcare expenses were borne by households. This figure is 55% in India and 54% in Pakistan.

These statistics indicate fewer opportunities for the medical treatment of victims of the infection and place a higher premium on prevention efforts. The lack of governmental medical reach may also mean that we can expect the public to rely less on the advice of the government about their personal health.

Despite a similarly low reach, the healthcare systems in the three countries differ in how they are administered. Bangladesh's healthcare system is highly centralized. The Ministry of Health and Family Welfare manages larger hospitals and community clinics, while the Ministry of Local Government, Rural Development and Cooperatives manages the provision of primary care services in urban areas (World Health Organization, 2015). In addition to the public healthcare providers, Bangladesh has a large number of private-sector healthcare providers.

In India and Pakistan, the responsibility for healthcare provision is shared among regional and central governments. Schedule 7 of the Constitution of India, which describes the jurisdictions of the federal government and states, allocates public health and health care to states ("6. Public health and sanitation; hospitals and dispensaries"). According to article 47 of the Constitution, "the State shall regard the raising of the level of nutrition and the standard of living of its people and the improvement of public health as among its primary duties." Schedule 4 of the Constitution of Pakistan lists the areas of exclusive federal and concurrent jurisdictions, with the remaining powers allocated to provinces (article 142 of the Constitution of Pakistan; 18th Amendment). The healthcare is not included in either list and, thus, falls within the jurisdiction of the subnational governments.

In practice, both states and union territories in India and provinces of Pakistan carry out the day-to-day administration of hospitals and the healthcare system. In both countries, the federal government has a coordinating and macro-regulatory role, both in regular healthcare provision and crisis response. While both countries have national ministries of health (the Union Ministry of Health and Family Welfare in India and the

Ministry of National Health Services, Regulation and Coordination in Pakistan), their responsibilities are limited to determining the overall health policy and running nationwide programs.

4.3.3 Epidemic Response Powers

Much like healthcare provision, the responsibility and powers to respond to an infectious disease outbreak in India and Pakistan are, according to their legal frameworks, shared by federal and subnational governments.

The *Epidemic Diseases Act of* 1897 was introduced to tackle the bubonic plague epidemic that had broken out in Bombay, and its broader aim was to prevent the spread of "dangerous epidemic diseases" (*Epidemic Diseases Act* 1897). The version of the act in effect in present-day India grants special powers to state authorities to implement special measures to curb the spread of contagious diseases. This one-page law consists of four sections, each dealing with, briefly, (1) the title and extent of the act, (2) empowering states to implement mitigating measures and to inspect and quarantine persons suspected of being infected and grants the central government to inspect and quarantine ships and their crew, (3) prescribing penalties for violating these regulations in accordance with Section 188 of the Indian Penal Code, and (4) guaranteeing legal protection to the officials implementing these policies.

Pakistan has also inherited a version of the Epidemic Diseases Act of 1897. The 1958 Epidemic Diseases Act for West Pakistan is essentially the same law with a modified name, i.e., Pakistan instead of India. At the time, all provinces of West Pakistan were treated as a single unit, and after East Pakistan became independent in 1971, the law applied to the rest of Pakistan. After the 18th Amendment to the Constitution of Pakistan (2010) gave provinces the responsibility for public health provision, the provincial governments replicated this law to be able to access the powers necessary for an epidemic response (e.g., Sindh Epidemic Diseases Act 2014).

In Bangladesh, the primary document governing epidemic response is the Infectious Diseases (Prevention, Control and Elimination) Act of 2018. While the country did inherit the Epidemic Diseases Act of 1897, it was replaced in 2018 with more extensive legislation. This law was formulated around the dengue epidemic with significant participation of the WHO. It gave considerable emergency powers to the health ministry and the national government.

4.3.4 Disaster Management Regulations

During the pandemic, all three countries invoked recently established national systems for national disaster planning and management.

The Indian National Disaster Management Authority (NDMA) was established under the Disaster Management Act of 2005, and its role was further elaborated in the National Policy on Disaster Management of 2009 and the National Disaster Management Plan of 2019. The act was created as a formal institutional mechanism for a national response to disasters, which had historically fallen within the purview of state governments (Ray 2005; Sarkar and Sarma 2005). The act defined a disaster as a "… catastrophe, mishap, calamity or grave occurrence in any area, arising from natural or man made causes, or by accident or negligence …" Missing from this definition is mention of disease epidemics. Similarly, "disaster management" was defined as "… a continuous and integrated process of planning, organizing, and implementing measures …" The act also provided for the creation of national-, state-, and district-level disaster management plans and established the NDMA with the prime minister of India as chairperson and up to nine members nominated by him or her, as well as a National Executive Committee (NEC) with the union home secretary as chairperson and the secretaries to various ministries and departments within the government of India and the chief of the Integrated Defense Staff of the Chiefs of Staff Committee as members. In addition to the national authority, the act created parallel state- and district-level disaster management bodies. It also outlined the role of subdistrict-level authorities for managing disasters, carrying out relief, rehabilitation, and reconstruction activities in the affected areas and the role of the National Disaster Response Force (NDRF) in assisting with disaster relief. The act stipulates that the NEC will coordinate the response to any disaster and outlines the roles and responsibilities of other bodies. The act also provides for the use of emergency powers in such situations and defines penalties for obstruction, noncompliance, misinformation, and abuse.

The National Disaster Management Plan of 2019, adopted under the aforementioned act, included major infectious disease outbreaks under the rubric of "Biological and Public Health Emergencies" and specified the roles of various government agencies (primarily at the level of the federal government) in surveillance, data collection and dissemination, training, and procurement. Importantly, while the Epidemic Diseases Act—much like public health regulations in more normal times—puts the onus of responsibility on state governments, the disaster management system in India reserves the leading role in epidemic response for the federal government.

The Pakistani NDMA was established under the National Disaster Management Ordinance of 2006 in the aftermath of the 2005 Kashmir earthquake. This ordinance took India's Disaster Management Act of 2005 as a model and was transformed by the national parliament into the National Disaster Management Act of 2010 in December 2010. The ordinance and act provided for the creation of national-, provincial-, and district-level disaster management plans and established bodies similar to those in India: a NDMA with an appointed director general as chairperson and a NEC (not to be confused with the committee) with the prime minister of Pakistan as chairperson, leader of the opposition in the Senate and National Assembly, various federal cabinet ministers, chief ministers of all provinces as well as the prime minister of AJ&K, chairman of the Joint Chiefs of Staff Committee or his nominee, and a representative of civil society or any other person nominated by the prime minister. In addition to national bodies, the act created parallel Provincial Disaster Management Authorities (PDMAs) and District Disaster Management Authorities (DDMAs). It also outlined the role of subdistrict-level authorities for managing disasters, carrying out relief, rehabilitation, and reconstruction activities in affected areas. The act stipulates that the federal government will coordinate the response to any disaster and outlines the roles and responsibilities of other bodies to whom it reserves more extensive responsibilities for subnational authorities. The act also provides for the use of emergency powers in such situations and defines penalties for obstruction, noncompliance, misinformation, and abuse. The definition of disaster in this act falls short of classifying epidemic diseases as a disaster.

What stands out despite the unavoidable similarity between the two acts is that Pakistan's National Disaster Management Act of 2010 includes more actors, including opposition and civil society members on commissions. Moreover, Pakistan's NDMA has a dedicated director general appointed by the prime minister usually from in-service army officers. Bangladesh's

Disaster Management Act of 2012 provides for the establishment of a National Disaster Management Council (NDMC) with the prime minister of Bangladesh as chairperson, various cabinet ministers, armed forces chiefs, sectaries of various ministries and departments, and the chairman of the National Disaster Management Advisory Committee. The act provided for the creation of a National Disaster Management Policy and National Disaster Management Plan. Unlike the disaster management systems in India and Pakistan, Bangladesh has a permanent Department of Disaster Management, which acts as the principal body for the coordination and conduct of disaster relief as well as implementation of National Disaster Management Policy and National Disaster Management Plans. The Disaster Management Act also provides for the formation of a National Disaster Response Coordination Group with the Minister of Food and Disaster Management as chairperson, Minister of Local Government, Rural Development and Cooperation, the principal staff officer of the Armed Forces Division, and sectaries of various ministries and departments to evaluate disaster situations and coordinate a response, as well as a national-level disaster management committee and local-level disaster management committee and group. The act provides for the use of emergency powers as well as military assets in disaster areas and defines penalties for obstruction, noncompliance, misinformation, and the abuse of the vested authority.

One point that distinguishes the disaster management system in Bangladesh from its counterparts in India and Pakistan is the fact that its founding act classifies pandemics and contagion as disasters. Even though the disaster management systems were used in all three countries during the COVID-19 pandemic, only in Bangladesh are health crises included in the jurisdictions of this system in the legislated disaster management document.

Table 4.2 summarizes the features of the organization of healthcare provision and disaster management by country.

4.4   COVID-19 Policy Response in 2020

4.4.1   Overview

According to confirmed case counts, COVID-19 reached India in January 2020, Pakistan in February 2020, and Bangladesh in March 2020. As Figure 4.1 shows, over the course of that year, all three countries saw the first major wave of the pandemic. Major upsurges started in mid to late March, with the new case counts reaching their peaks in June in Bangladesh and Pakistan and in September in India.

Figure 4.1 also shows a silhouette of the government and community responses to the outbreak. The overall stringency of nonmedical

86   A. B. ADEEL AND A. ZHIRNOV

Table 4.2 Differences in health crisis response structures in India, Pakistan, and Bangladesh

Country	Constitutional responsibility for health care	Healthcare devolution	Disaster management body	Latest rules on disaster management
India	Yes	Federal (limited) + regional (proactive)	National Disaster Management Authority (2005)	National Disaster Management Plan (2019)
Pakistan	No	Federal (limited) + regional (proactive)	National Disaster Management Authority (2006)	National Disaster Management Act (2010)
Bangladesh	Yes	Central government	Department of Disaster Management (2012)	Disaster Management Act (2012)

interventions is captured using the average total Protective Policy Index (Shvetsova et al. 2022). This index takes into account both subnational and national policies across fifteen categories of nonmedical targeted and indiscriminate measures.

The panel "Community Mobility" relies on Google Community Mobility reports (Google LLC, 2020). These reports contain information about the foot traffic in the retail and recreational areas, at workplaces, transit stations, and grocery stores, as well as the amount of time spent in residential areas. All indicators are computed as a percent change relative to the values of these statistics in January-February 2020. The value shown in Figure 4.1 is the average change in mobility along the aforementioned dimensions (following Van Bavel et al., 2020).

The similarity in the trajectories of both the overall policy stringency and the community response, particularly at the outset of the lockdowns, is striking. Figure 4.1 reveals a significant increase in policy stringency and a corresponding significant drop in policy stringency in late March 2020. Indeed, around March 22 to 24, all three countries initiated a version of a lockdown and introduced a number of accompanying measures, which can serve as a critical event separating phases 1 and 2 in our narrative. The public responded by radically reducing their activities outside of

4 COVID-19 RESPONSE IN INDIA, PAKISTAN, AND BANGLADESH: SHARED... 87

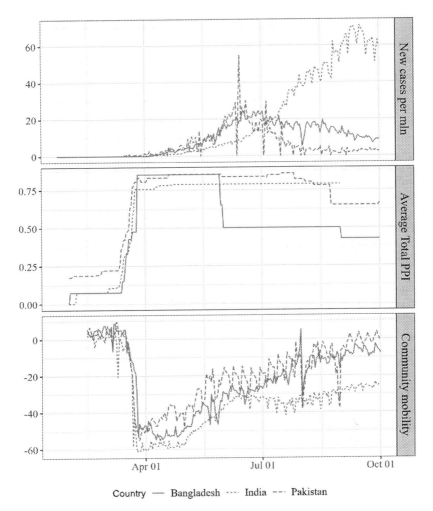

Fig. 4.1 Dynamics of infection outbreak and policy response in India, Pakistan, and Bangladesh, 2020. (Source: Shvetsova et al. 2022)

residential areas, with some activities slowly revitalized starting early May. In mid-May, the governments started lifting the restrictions.

In what follows, we discuss the process by which the aforementioned actors produced those outcomes. Despite the similarities in policy outcomes, we will see striking differences in the process that led to them.

The discussion of the COVID-19 policy response in 2020, at least in South Asia, can be best broken down into discussions of three phases. Figure 4.2 defines those phases based on the data at hand the earlier outlined taxonomy of public health measures.

According to this schema, initially, the activities are limited to on-demand medical assistance to infected individuals. Phase 1 is when governments attempt to isolate potential nodes of infection spread. If those

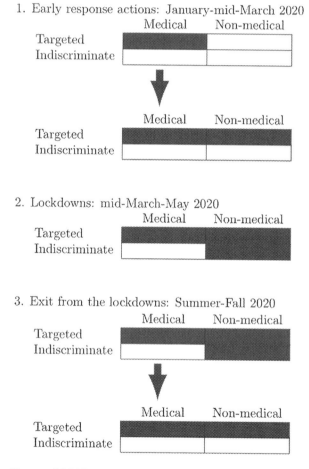

Fig. 4.2 Phases of COVID-19 pandemic response in 2020

measures fail to stop community spread, as was the case in the COVID-19 pandemic, governments may move to broad restrictions reducing the density of in-person interactions in the community at large (phase 2). Phase 3 is the gradual lifting of those restrictions. Since vaccines were not available at that time, mass vaccination was not an option.

4.4.2 Phase I in India

The first phase saw preemptive and containment measures taken by state and national governments. The Indian central government started regular meetings on potential actions to take in response to the COVID-19 outbreak in mid-January 2020 while issuing action recommendations to state governments. It acted through the NDMA—an emergency body led, ex officio, by the prime minister and coordinating the actions of the relevant central and state government agencies. Under the current disaster management plan (National Disaster Management Plan 2019), COVID-19 fell under the rubric of "Biological and Public Health Emergencies." Since the plan concerned itself primarily with the areas of surveillance, data collection and dissemination, training, and medical capacity building, these were the areas that featured most in the initial NDMA communications.

Parallel to that, we see the application of border closures across India and other cross-border containment measures. Kerala became the first state to announce self-isolation policy for incomers with recent travel to China starting February 3,[1] followed by Andhra Pradesh the next day. This was supplemented by suspending visas with China and issuing a quarantine recommendation by the national government on February 7— almost a week later than Pakistan implemented similar measures. The national government extended similar visa restrictions to other hotspots including Iran, Italy, and South Korea, a month later on March 3. Even more stringent and mandatory quarantine measures were introduced on March 12. Arunachal Pradesh became the first to ban foreign tourists from entry to stop the spread on March 8, followed by Himachal Pradesh on March 18, Uttarakhand on March 20, and Goa on 21 March. The national government also closed borders with neighboring countries Nepal, Bhutan, Bangladesh, and Myanmar on March 15.

---

[1] For the sources of this information, see the changes file in the Protective Policy Index dataset (Shvetsova et al. 2022).

On February 26, the Ministry of Health and Family Affairs circulated a plan for cluster containment, which delegated the actual implementation of containment zones to states and districts. On March 11, the central government recommended all state governments to invoke Section 2 of the Epidemic Diseases Act of 1897, thereby assuming additional powers necessary to implement strict containment protocols, such as sealing affected areas, criminalizing social gatherings, and implementing mandatory quarantines, among others, and most states obliged. On March 14, the central government declared COVID-19 a notified disaster, granting affected areas access to disaster funds.

While we see that the efforts of the central government can lead state- and district-level actions to halt community spread of a virus (and, it would seem, to delay more stringent measures), there is also evidence of some subnational actions ahead of those of the federal government. Andhra Pradesh became the first state to implement strict social gathering protocols (Section 144 banning gatherings of five or more people) in some of its districts as early as March 4. Section 144 was later imposed in Bihar on March 14, in Chhattisgarh on March 20, and Kerala and Maharashtra on March 22. The Delhi government was the first to close primary schools on March 5, followed by the closure of all schools, colleges, and universities on March 12. Karnataka also closed primary schools on March 9 after the first case in the state was confirmed and all other institutes on the next day. Others followed suit: Rajasthan, Odisha, Uttar Pradesh, Bihar, and Chhattisgarh closed their schools on March 13, followed by Punjab, Haryana, Himachal Pradesh, Maharashtra, Madhya Pradesh, and Goa on March 14; Assam and Gujarat on March 15; Jharkhand and West Bengal on March 16; and Arunachal Pradesh, Mizoram, and Nagaland on March 17. Such orders were also accompanied by closures of other crowded places such as malls, cinemas, theaters, gyms, and swimming pools, as well as restrictions on social gatherings and sporting events. There was a gradual reduction in the number of people allowed to gather for weddings/funerals and other events.

4.4.3   *Phase I in Pakistan*

In Pakistan, the health authorities had the responsibility for the original response. Its National Institute of Health was the first agency to respond to the possibility of the COVID-19 spreading in the country. In January

2020, its Field Epidemiology and Disease Surveillance Division issued two advisories—one for travelers and another for medical professionals.

Similar to (and likely to a greater extent than) India, cross-border containment was a major priority in the policy response. The earliest steps in COVID-19 response in Pakistan were taken in Gilgit-Baltistan, the territory bordering China. The local government requested that the center delay opening the land border—Khubnjrab Pass, the main trade route to and from China—to curb potential spillover on January 27 (and the federal government complied). The federal government of Pakistan suspended flights from China on January 31 and declared a mandatory quarantine condition for returnees from China on February 1. However, it was not China but Iran and, to a certain degree, Saudi Arabia, home to holy sites of Shia and Sunni Muslims, that became the transmission route to Pakistan. The mode of transmission apparently was pilgrimage (Badshah et al. 2020), rather than recreational tourism, as was the case in India and many other West European countries. Meanwhile, the federal government also implemented thermal screening procedures on airports starting February 2, and the National Institute of Health started providing assistance and guidelines to establish provincial surveillance units.

The northerwestern province, Khyber Pakhtunkhwa, took the lead in declaring an emergency on February 4, citing the need to quarantine travelers. Other provinces followed suit, with Baluchistan declaring an emergency on February 23. Provincial authorities in the southwestern province, Baluchistan, which shares a border with the regional hub Iran, cordoned off the land border on February 24 and stopped pilgrims from Iran from entering the province. Later on, quarantine centers were established at the border to screen incomers from Iran, who were then transported inland to different centers in other provinces. Other border closures were ordered by the federal government: the border with Afghanistan was sealed on March 1 following the confirmation of the first COVID-19 case in Afghanistan.

School closures started in Baluchistan, the province bordering Iran, and Sindh, where the megapolis of Karachi is located; these governments closed schools, colleges, and universities on February 27, followed by Khyber Pakhtunkhwa on March 13. Punjab announced a medical emergency on March 12, Gilgit-Baltistan also on March 12, Sindh on March 14, and Azad Kashmir on March 16. Meanwhile, the center and provinces also scrambled to curb social gatherings, and Section 144 was imposed in many places to discourage gatherings of five or more people. The Indo-Pak border was closed on March 19, and all air travel was closed on March 22.

On March 13, the National Security Committee, which deals largely with international security threats, held its first ever meeting on a public health matter. It confirmed the closure of the western border, school closures, and the cancellation of large public gatherings. The same day, the National Institute of Health issued a National Action Plan establishing an emergency core committee. The plan allocated tasks to various agencies of the federal government, and, to a lesser degree, to the provincial governments. It focused on containment and risk communication measures at the time.

4.4.4 Phase I in Bangladesh

In Bangladesh, the Institute of Epidemiology, Disease Control and Research was initially tasked with leading the coronavirus response; however, most actions were announced at the meetings of the cabinet of ministers. The first actions in response to the COVID-19 outbreak prioritized the prevention of imported cases. The government started screening all arrivals on January 22. On February 2, the government of Bangladesh decided to stop granting on-arrival visas for Chinese visitors until further notice and sealed its border with Myanmar; it suspended on-arrival visas for all countries on March 14. Starting March 16, the government called for fourteen-day quarantines for all new arrivals. Starting March 17, the government closed educational institutions, and on March 19 the government prohibited mass gatherings and empowered the military to help division and district officials to enforce those actions.

4.4.5 Phase II (Lockdowns)

All three countries—India, Pakistan, and Bangladesh—imposed national lockdowns during the week of March 23, as shown in Figure 4.3.

In India, the first country-wide lockdown was initiated, as a trial run, by Prime Minister Modi on March 22 under the name of "Janata curfew": the people ("Janata") were urged not to leave their homes for a day. On March 24, the Ministry of Home Affairs, on behalf of the NDMA, issued

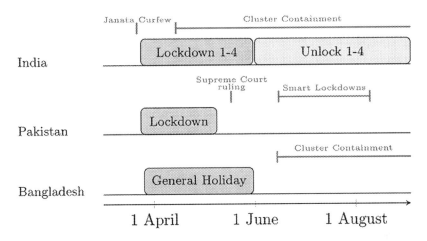

Fig. 4.3 Timing of national lockdowns in India, Pakistan, and Bangladesh. (Source: Shvetsova et al. 2022)

an order and guidelines for the implementation of a three-week nationwide lockdown. These guidelines listed the actions to be taken by state governments and the administrations of union territories (UTs), including the types of establishments and venues allowed to stay open and those being forced to close, restrictions on the movement of persons and gatherings, and other measures. It was the responsibility of subnational governments—empowered by the Epidemic Diseases Act of 1897—to issue lockdown orders and implement them.

It is under these powers that select states initiated lockdowns prior to the "orders" of the central government. Delhi, Bihar, and Odisha announced a comprehensive lockdown on March 21, followed by Madhya Pradesh, Rajasthan, Punjab, Himachal Pradesh, Mizoram, Haryana on March 22, and Arunachal Pradesh, Assam, Gujarat, and Goa on March 23.

In Pakistan, after initial calls for social distancing and self-isolation, one after another the provinces started implementing strict lockdown measures. Azad Kashmir closed its domestic borders and ordered a ban on public transport on March 17, followed by a lockdown the following day. Sindh went into lockdown on March 20, followed by Gilgit-Baltistan on March 22, Punjab on March 23, Baluchistan on March 24, and Islamabad on March 25. Before that, various provinces had dabbled with partial measures like closing malls, restricting public transport, shutting down

94 A. B. ADEEL AND A. ZHIRNOV

eateries, and sealing off parks, among others. However, ultimately lockdowns were implemented.

The national government joined efforts to enforce the restrictions with a delay. While Pakistani Prime Minister Khan expressed reluctance to implement a national lockdown, on March 24 military spokesman Major General Iftikhar announced that the military would oversee it. On March 28, the National Coordination Committee created the National Command and Operation Center (NCOC) to coordinate the efforts of military and civilian personnel. Around the same time, on March 26, the federal health ministry issued guidelines for social distancing, which recommended that residents stay at home except for essential travel.

In Bangladesh, a lockdown was announced on March 22 (to start on March 26) under the name of "general holiday." The general holiday required the closures of private and public offices, imposed restrictions on public transportation and interdistrict movement, prohibited mass gatherings, and set limits on the movement of residents. The lockdown was strictly enforced with the involvement of police and the army.

4.4.6 Phase III (exit from broad lockdowns and cluster containment)

In India, the exit from the national lockdown started in mid-April. The strategy was based on the idea of identifying areas of outbreak, restricting people's movement between those areas and the outside, and allowing a gradual lifting of restrictions everywhere else.

On April 14, the government issued guidelines for Lockdown 2.0, which included a classification of the country's districts into red, orange, and green. The classification was based on the dynamics of cases and was set up by the federal health ministry. At the time, there were 170 red zone districts, 207 orange, and 359 green zone districts. The rules allowed state governments to relax lockdown orders in select sectors (healthcare, agricultural, financial sectors) starting April 20; however, such relaxation was not allowed in red zone districts.

As most state governments were reluctant to relax the rules outside of red zones (e.g., Jharkhand and Bihar did not relax restrictions at all) and ease the pressure for the national government to keep lifting the restrictions (or at least keep announcing them), the definition of hot zones was gradually handed over to state governments. On May 1, Lockdown 3.0 enabled state governments to lower the status of the district defined by the federal health ministry (make an orange district red) and designate specific parts of red districts as orange (e.g., rural parts of predominantly urban districts). State governments could also identify containment zones within red and orange districts. In cities, containment zones could cover just a ward or a municipal zone. Soon, the containment zones approach superseded the classification of districts. Starting with Lockdown 4.0 (May 17), the containment zones were defined solely by state governments.

On June 1, the central government declared the start of the end of lockdowns and initiated the so-called Unlock 1.0 phase, followed by Unlock 2.0, Unlock 3.0, and so on until the end of the year. These guidelines suggested that the state governments may choose to lift classes of restrictions outside of containment zones, which were also defined by state governments.

In Pakistan, the easing of the lockdown started in mid-April by the decision of the national government to lift restrictions from select industries. On April 18, the federal government, without consulting the provincial governments, agreed to reopen mosques across the country. On May 9, the prime minister announced the decision of the National Coordination Committee to replace the strict version of the lockdown with a "partial" lockdown. Schools and public transportation remained closed, but small markets in residential areas and shops and most construction, agriculture, paper, and other companies in "lower-risk" industries were allowed to open.

When the Sindh government objected, a *suo moto* ruling of the Supreme Court upheld the federal government's decision and directed the Sindh government to comply. On May 18, the Supreme Court declared that the coronavirus was "not a pandemic in Pakistan" and directed the reopening of shopping centers in the dissenting Sindh province.

In mid-June, after the onset of a new spike in cases and WHO appeals, the NCOC directed the implementation of a "smart lockdown" ("tracing, testing, and quarantine" strategy): the closing-up of local containment zones. The areas of concern were identified by the federal government; however, it was provincial governments whose orders established the containment zones. According to the Pakistani newspaper *Dawn*, there were 904 containment zones in Punjab, 572 in Khyber Pakhtunkhwa, 29 in Azad Kashmir, 26 in Sindh, 10 in Islamabad, and 5 in Gilgit-Baltistan. "Smart lockdowns" would be removed on August 10.

In Bangladesh, the initial "general holiday" lasted until May 27. After that, most of the restrictions were lifted, although gatherings were still banned, and there remained restrictions on transportation and interdistrict movement. Schools remained closed until the end of the year.

Similarly to India and Pakistan, the relaxation of restrictions in Bangladesh was accompanied by the creation of cluster containment zones. On June 12, the ministry of health (specifically, the Directorate General of Health Services) introduced a zone-based containment strategy. It identified red, yellow, and green zones according to the severity of the outbreak. The lockdown rules persisted in red zones, which were fenced off from green zones. The responsibility for the implementation of these measures was borne by city corporations and district administrations; however, the army helped enforce these measures.

4.4.7 How Formal Powers Were Used during the Pandemic

As promised in Section 4.2, here we draw some conclusions about the trajectories of the COVID-19 policy response in the three countries under consideration and the roles of different governments in the formulation of that response.

As the preceding discussion shows, the overall trajectories of the policies and the community response were very similar. Governments were reluctant to implement strict community-wide restrictions and, once they implemented them, could manage to effectively maintain those restrictions only for two months. In mid to late May they started lifting the restrictions, albeit with different degrees of gradualism. The further subsequent surge of cases forced them to adopt a system of cluster containment zones, which offered a localized alternative to comprehensive restrictions.

Both India and Pakistan are federations, and, as we have seen, their laws and regulations contain similar allocations of responsibilities for healthcare provision and epidemic response. Their regional governments are uniquely empowered to implement epidemic-related restrictions (and, being responsible for the operation of public healthcare systems, have fiscal pressures to do so). The national governments are empowered by disaster management frameworks to coordinate healthcare provision and epidemic response. Despite similarities in the countries' respective legal frameworks, interactions between federal and subnational governments worked in different ways in these two countries.

In India, the disaster management system was effectively used by the federal government to coordinate the actions of the state governments through bureaucratic and intergovernmental channels. It is hard to say whether the state governments would have adopted completely different measures in the absence of the disaster management system and the involvement of the federal government, but there is evidence that some state governments felt their hand was forced around the introduction of the lockdowns. Even though they lacked the resources to implement them, they were compelled to do so by the federal government's announcement, leading to tensions in intergovernmental relations (Tremblay and George 2021). As the federal government reduced its involvement in the formulation of nonmedical intervention policies in May-June and state governments recovered effective agency in pandemic measures, we saw greater variation in the emerging local public health regimes without significant intergovernmental conflicts.

In Pakistan, there was significant involvement of ad hoc actors and visible intergovernmental conflicts over the pandemic response. Epidemic disease acts were invoked by provincial governments to initiate lockdowns and produce other nonmedical interventions, much like in India. This, however, met initially with resistance from the federal government. But the disaster management authority did not engage in policy coordination and served primarily as a centralized procurement authority. Despite the presence of NDMA to coordinate disaster management efforts between federal and provincial governments in Pakistan, a new body named the NCOC was established in April 2020 to coordinate the response to the COVID-19 pandemic. NCOC executives included a federal minister and a lieutenant general of the Pakistani army. This institutional ambiguity created confusion among stakeholders that was noticed by the media (Tanzeem 2020). The military was involved in the major decisions around the formulation of a national COVID-19 response, including the decision to enforce lockdown rules with the assistance of the army. Another somewhat unexpected participant in the formulation of COVID-19 policies was the Supreme Court, which sided with the federal government as it faced resistance from the Sindh government during the lifting of lockdowns.

4.5 Looking for the Antecedent of COVID-19 Responses in History

To try to understand these differences in the actual interplay between federal and subnational governments in India and Pakistan, as well as the haste with which the government moved from broad community-wide mitigation strategies to cluster containment, we resort to a historical institutional analysis of the current frameworks.

98   A. B. ADEEL AND A. ZHIRNOV

4.5.1   *Historicizing the Pandemic Response*

We argue in light of the theoretical framework described in what follows that existing institutional frameworks—their allowances and deficiencies—were the reasons we observed how the public health response was implemented in these countries. Their shared past somewhat dictated their present policies.

As new institutionalism theory suggests, political activity is limited by the institutional structures that actors create and within which they operate. Historical institutionalism as a branch of institutionalism concerns itself with continuity and change in formal and informal rules, norms, and procedures—i.e., institutions—embedded in organizational structures of a polity *over time*. Its primary analytical interest lies in explaining *institutional development*, i.e., "the construction, maintenance, and adaptation of institutions" (Sanders, 2006, p. 42). The simple governing logic is that institutions tend to persist once they are established until a critical juncture disturbs this order and necessitates a new arrangement.

Historical institutionalists also maintain that institutions alone are not the only causal force[2] (Hall & Taylor 1996, p. 942) and "hypothesize about the combined effects of institutions and processes" (Pierson & Skocpol, 2002, p. 696). Institutional development in the long run is marked by *path dependence*, i.e., subsequent events in a time sequence are not independent of antecedent conditions (Pierson 2000). It dictates that how new institutional forms emerge depends on the previous arrangements. Path dependence restricts the possibility of change as when a path becomes "well travelled," it becomes increasingly difficult to carve out a new one (Pierson 2000). Such path dependence is broken when crises or shocks hit, stipulating new ways of doing things. Such critical junctures are the bedrock of institutional development. *Critical junctures* are significant, system-level exogenous events or series of events that make dramatic change a real possibility (Capoccia & Kelemen, 2007). These perturbations act like a "switchman" that could potentially set institutions on a different path than the one they had been on before the perturbations.

We argue here that our understanding of the institutional response to COVID-19 in India, Pakistan, and Bangladesh might be incomplete without contextualizing the development of public health frameworks in general and this with regard to COVID-19 in particular in these countries.

---

[2] Institutions + path dependence + critical junctures + actors

Intergovernmental interaction at national and subnational levels and the resultant COVID-19 response can be traced back to how the British Raj managed state affairs and dealt with deadly pandemics during colonial times.

4.5.2 British India

The political development of the Indian subcontinent started as early as the 12th century BC. It saw the rise and decline of several empires (including the fabled Mughal Empire), uniting or almost uniting the region politically. India, Pakistan, and Bangladesh constituted a single state—the historical India—until 1947, which is when Pakistan separated on religious grounds, leading to a division of that single landmass into East and West Pakistan, flanked by India. East Pakistan then split off from West Pakistan—now simply Pakistan—on ethnic grounds to become Bangladesh in 1971. The development of the Weberian state—bureaucratic and legal-rational state—coincided with British domination of India, particularly the period of direct rule of the British Crown between 1858 and 1947.

The British Raj, as the British colonial administration was called, replaced the existing governance structures with Western style institutions starting with the Indian Civil Service, which replaced East India Company as the colonial administrator. The Raj also introduced an extensive legal framework rooted in common law tradition to facilitate India's direct integration into the British Empire (Dwivedi et al. 1989). India, Pakistan, and Bangladesh inherited this framework, which was readily integrated into the new constitutions—sometimes with minor amendments or mere name changes to reflect the postpartition reality. For example, The Indian Penal Code 1860 was instituted as Indian, Pakistan, and Bangladesh Penal Codes as criminal code of the land in these countries. As another example, all three countries inherited the Westminster system and first-past-the-post elections.

India and Pakistan also inherited their federal systems from the British Raj. The Government of India Act of 1935 heralded the independence of India and provided for the establishment of a Federation of India, which was later adopted by both India and Pakistan as the system of governance in both countries. Bangladesh, however, became a unitary state upon independence from Pakistan (it was a single province of East Pakistan right before declaring its independence).

4.5.3 Public Health in the British Raj

Figure 4.4 shows the major milestones in the development of epidemic response systems in the three countries. The history of modern outbreak response systems in British India started in the middle of the nineteenth century with the expansion of the municipal-level public health responsibilities in the major urban areas – just like in England – and the work of the Indian Medical Service and the Sanitary Department primarily for the civil service and the army (Jeffery, 1988; Harrison, 1994; Polu, 2012). The 1880s saw the codification of emergency public health powers in the charters of major cities.

The 1896–1900 bubonic plague epidemic is a critical junction that led to the making of the first government-level law for responding to outbreaks. When the epidemic hit Bombay in 1896 and the government faced increased pressure from abroad to increase the safety of goods through Indian ports, it adopted the Epidemic Diseases Act of 1897 (Gatacre 1897). This act was very short and almost word for word copied a section of the Bombay Municipal Charter, 1888 (See sections 412–441 and particularly Section 434) and gave emergency powers to the governor general

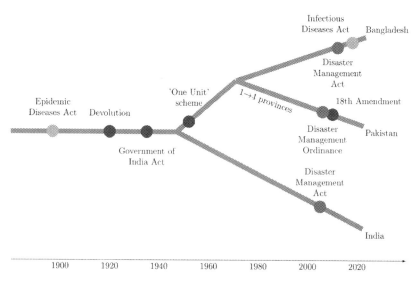

Fig. 4.4 Institutional trajectories of epidemic response systems in India, Pakistan, and Bangladesh

4 COVID-19 RESPONSE IN INDIA, PAKISTAN, AND BANGLADESH: SHARED... 101

in council (read colonial administration). The municipal plague committee, led by medical professionals, was replaced by governmental committees led by Brigadier General William Gatacre and the army with limited participation of the medical service. The plague committee was innovative with various public health measures and increased the stringency of the regime through 1897–1898; however, it met with resistance and had, by its own admission, limited knowledge of the disease (Harrison, 1994), and it was rather unsuccessful.

Responding to epidemics and enacting public health measures outside cities was even more difficult. Two features of the context of British India were particularly impactful. First, the government had a patchy presence in the country. Both the civil service and the army concentrated in or around major ports with limited presence inland. Second, sanitary conditions were difficult; there was limited infrastructure for clean water supplies and amenities.

Most of the diseases that would emerge in Europe from time to time and be considered epidemics were endemic in British India. The plague, first appearing in the 1890s, killed people in the interior of British India well into the 1930s (Public Health Commissioner with the Government of India 1941). Eradication of these diseases was considered impractical as they were, to a large degree, attributed to the climate and poor sanitary conditions and had limited influence on trade and economy (Amrith 2009; Arnold 1993). Medical methods – curative medicine and vaccination – were given priority over regular or emergency nonmedical interventions (Harrison 1994). As a consequence, researchers have observed an accelerated development of medical research in the subcontinent, but no comprehensive framework or tradition of public health mobilization or community-wide public health efforts.

Although it is beyond the scope of this chapter, it might be instructive to compare the development of the public health systems in former British India against their development in Canada. There, public health efforts were made at the municipal, provincial, and central levels alike and were partially driven by a broad public acceptance of the necessity of restrictions during and outside of outbreaks (e.g., Rutty and Sullivan 2010; Bielska et al. 2015).

Attempts to introduce such frameworks had limited success, in part due to the complexity of federal bargaining in India and Pakistan. Any comprehensive framework would have to couple epidemic responsibilities with emergency resources at the same level of government, which would require either shifting responsibilities away from subnational governments or granting them access to more financial and personnel resources at the expense of the federal government. As Amrith (2009) points out, the motivation to treat health as a right in postcolonial India faced a challenge in existing fiscal relations.

As discussed earlier, the Epidemic Diseases Act of 1897, which lacked specifics of the implementation of epidemic response and coordination with the healthcare system, remains the primary legal document for such a response in India and Pakistan and was only recently replaced in Bangladesh. In 2018, with major participation by the World Health Organization, it adopted the Infectious Diseases (Prevention, Control and Eradication) Act. The act is very detailed and provides for a clearer division of roles and communication among various agencies, including the public healthcare system. None of this should suggest that the division of roles and communication among agencies could not take place in India and Pakistan; however, there it took additional organizing efforts and political leadership.

4.5.4 Public Health Federalism

The original Epidemic Diseases Act of 1897 granted powers to the central governments, but the current versions of that act in India and Pakistan specifically grant powers to subnational governments. How did this happen, and what implications did it have for the COVID-19 response?

The Montague-Chelmsford reforms (1919) and the Government of India Act (1935) led to the devolution of public health responsibilities to provincial governments and corresponding amendments in the Epidemic Diseases Act. Following independence, India and Pakistan inherited the subnational-centered version of the act; however, due to the "One Unit" doctrine, power did not devolve below the level of the province of West Pakistan. Only after the 1973 constitution and, particularly, the 18th amendment adopted in 2010, did the provincial governments receive significant autonomy in the area.

In 2005 and 2006, respectively, India and Pakistan created disaster management and planning systems that gave the respective federal governments coordinating and planning roles in the management of disasters, which, though not intended originally, could be used during major outbreaks of infectious diseases and were invoked during the COVID-19 pandemic.

Despite the similarities between the settings, the interactions between federal and subnational governments in Pakistan followed very different patterns. In the absence of a comprehensive framework, the coordinating powers of the disaster management system were only effective in India, not in Pakistan, where disagreements over policies led to an overt intergovernmental conflict. We suspect that at least part of the success of the system is that its design followed the template created by the planning commissions and finance commissions. These systems were created in the mid-20th century (the planning commissions were still in existence when the disaster management framework was established); they included parallel federal- and state-level bodies and socialized public officials into particular modes of interaction across levels of government. The disaster management system was built to carve out a role for the federal government in disaster response, which had previously been largely in the hands of state governments. The provision of parallel national- and state-level bodies and plans was arguably a way to apply a known institutional approach to yet another problem of intergovernmental relations at the time and, as a result, was relatively effective during the pandemic.

In contrast, in Pakistan, a disaster management system was established in 2006, before the major devolution of responsibilities to provinces (and before democratization). At the time the disaster management framework was created, public health was not yet the sole purview of provincial governments, and there had been no significant tradition of bureaucratic communication across levels of government. There was, however, a tradition of military involvement in emergency response and civil affairs, which helped to bridge the gap in intergovernmental communication.

4.6 MAKING SENSE OF THE PANDEMIC RESPONSE IN SOUTH ASIA

We have described how the public health response to the COVID-19 pandemic was implemented in India, Pakistan, and Bangladesh and found both similarities in the overall trajectory of the policy approach and significant differences in the formulation of those policies. All three countries implemented lockdowns in late March, started relaxing them after a while, and used technically similar approaches—built around the idea of cluster containment—to replace them. The politics were quite different. Bangladeshi policies were decided, with the active participation of health authorities, by the national government without visible internal differences regarding the appropriate strategy. Policymaking in India and

Pakistan—two federations—was shared by the national and subnational governments, but in different ways. Pakistan saw an overt conflict erupt between the federal and provincial governments over strategies, which was resolved through the participation of third-party actors—the military and the judiciary. Intergovernmental relations over COVID-19 policies in India, where the subnational and federal governments had their differences in preferences, were driven by well-instrumented bargaining.

It is hard to say to what degree the similarities in pandemic strategies were due to the common institutional legacy and to what degree they were due to similarities in the structural conditions—such as the prevalence of daily wage workers and manual work, poverty, distrust toward government, and rurality—and the sharing of policy templates across countries or through the WHO. That said, it does appear that the lack of a democratic political tradition (and a *political*—not just policy — framework) of an epidemic response contributed to the difficulties associated with maintaining public health restrictions long enough.

It is also fair to state that the lack of a political framework specific to a public health response contributed to the high degree to which the differences in the politics outside of public health shaped the formulation of the crisis response (also see Rakesh, 2016). It does not appear that the rules of public health response gave sufficient guidance to the governments in the federations about how to resolve their differences in preferences over the course of action and coordination. The lack of such a political framework is what allowed political factors, such as methods of political interaction across levels of government and the power of the judiciary and the army, to assert themselves. The COVID-19 pandemic represents, undeniably, a critical juncture and an opportunity to overhaul this severely deficient institutional framework, which we hope will lead to better institutions in this area.

References

Adeel AB et al (2020) COVID-19 policy response and the rise of the sub-national governments. Canadian Public Policy /Analyse de politique 46(4):565–584

Amrith SS (2009) Health in India since Independence. Number 79. In: BWPI Working Paper, Brooks World Poverty Institute.

Arnold D (1993) Colonizing the body: State medicine and epidemic disease in nineteenth century India. Oxford University Press, Delhi

Badshah SL, Ullah A, Badshah SH, & Ahmad I (2020) Spread of Novel coronavirus by returning pilgrims from Iran to Pakistan. Journal of Travel Medicine 27(3)

4 COVID-19 RESPONSE IN INDIA, PAKISTAN, AND BANGLADESH: SHARED... 105

Benton JE (2020) Challenges to federalism and intergovernmental relations and takeaways amid the COVID-19 experience. The American Review of Public Administration 50(6–7):536–542

Bielska IA et al (2015) Public health in Canada: An overview. Zdrowie Publiczne i Zarządzanie 13(2):165–179

Capoccia G, Kelemen R F (2007) The study of critical junctures: Theory, narrative, and counterfactuals in historical institutionalism. World Politics 59(3):341–369

Dwivedi OP, Jain RB, Dua BD (1989) Imperial legacy, bureaucracy, and administrative changes: India 1947–1987. Public Administration & Development (1986–1998) 9(3):253

Epidemic Diseases Act, (1897)

Gatacre W (1897) Report on the Bubonie plague in Bombay 1896–97. Times of India Steam Press, Bombay

Google LLC (2020) Google COVID-19 Community Mobility Reports. https://www.google.com/covid19/mobility/. Accessed 1 April 2021

Hall PA, Taylor RC (1996). Political science and the three new institutionalisms. Political Studies 44(5): 936–957.

Harrison M (1994) Public Health in British India: Anglo-Indian Preventive Medicine 1859–1914. Cambridge University Press, Cambridge.

Jeffery R (1988) The Politics of Health in India. University of California Press, Berkeley.

Lecours A et al. (2021) Explaining Intergovernmental Conflict in the COVID-19 Crisis: The United States, Canada, and Australia. Publius: The Journal of Federalism 51(4): 513–536

Pierson P (2000) Increasing returns, path dependence, and the study of politics. American Political Science Review 94(2):251–267

Pierson P, Skocpol T (2002). Historical institutionalism in contemporary political science. Political Science: The State of the Discipline 3(1):1–32

Polu SL (2012) Infectious Disease in India, 1892–1940: Policy-Making and the Perception of Risk. Palgrave Macmillan, Basingstoke

Public Health Commissioner with the Government of India (1941) Annual Report of Public Health Commissioner with the Government of India for 1940. Delhi: Manager of Publications.

Rakesh PS (2016) The epidemic diseases act of 1897: Public health relevance in the current scenario. Indian J Med Ethics 1(3):156–160

Ray CN (2005) A Note on the Disaster Management Bill, 2005. Economic and Political Weekly 40(47):4877–4881

Rutty C, Sullivan SC (2010) This is public health: A Canadian history. Public Health, 4(10)

Sanders E (2006) Historical Institutionalism. In: Rhodes RA, Binder SA, Rockman BA (eds) The Oxford Handbook of Political Institutions. Oxford University Press, Oxford

Schnabel J, Hegele Y (2021) Explaining intergovernmental coordination during the COVID-19 pandemic: Responses in Australia, Canada, Germany, and Switzerland. Publius: The Journal of Federalism 51(4): 537–569

Shvetsova O et al (2021) Federal Institutions and Strategic Policy Responses to COVID-19 Pandemic. Frontiers in Political Science 3:66

Shvetsova O et al (2022) Protective Policy Index (PPI) global dataset of origins and stringency of COVID 19 mitigation policies. Scientific Data 9(1):1–10

Tanzeem A (2020) Lockdown or No Lockdown? Confusion Dominates Pakistan's COVID Response. Voice of America (VOA). https://www.voanews.com/a/covid-19-pandemic_lockdown-or-no-lockdown-confusion-dominates-pakistans-covid-response/6188541.html. Accessed 14 September 2021

Tremblay RC, George N (2021) India: Federalism, majoritarian nationalism, and the vulnerable and marginalized. In: Ramraj VV (ed) Covid-19 in Asia: Law and Policy Contexts. Oxford University Press, Oxford, p 173–188

Van Bavel JJ et al (2020) National identity predicts public health support during a global pandemic. Nature Communications 13(1):1–14

Wibbels E (2005). *Federalism and the market: Intergovernmental conflict and economic reform in the developing world.* Cambridge University Press

World Health Organization (2015) Bangladesh health system review. WHO Regional Office for the Western Pacific. https://apps.who.int/iris/handle/10665/208214. Accessed 14 September 2021

World Health Organization (n.d.-a) Global Health Expenditure Database. https://apps.who.int/nha/database/ViewData/Indicators/en. Accessed 14 September 2021

World Health Organization (n.d.-b) The Global Health Observatory. Hospital beds (per 10000 population). https://www.who.int/data/gho/data/indicators/indicator-details/GHO/. Accessed 14 September 2021

CHAPTER 5

Center-Regional Political Risk Sharing in the COVID-19 Public Health Crisis: Nigeria and South Africa

Onsel Gurel Bayrali

5.1 Introduction

The COVID-19 pandemic has enabled social scientists to explore once again how political factors shape incumbents' incentives while sharing their intergovernmental responsibilities during the policymaking process in decentralized countries. COVID-19 restrictive measures as risky collective goods make the risk management process during task sharing in the fight against the pandemic more complicated. Risky collective goods refer to public goods provided at the regional or local level and pose a political (e.g., electoral) threat to their providers (political incumbents). Restrictive measures to combat coronavirus were such "risky collective goods."

Precautions to lessen the catastrophic impacts of pandemics are a double-edged sword for decision makers. The fast-spreading virus

---

O. G. Bayrali (✉)
Department of Political Science, Binghamton University,
Binghamton, NY, USA
e-mail: obayral1@binghamton.edu

© The Author(s), under exclusive license to Springer Nature Switzerland AG 2023
O. Shvetsova (ed.), *Government Responses to the COVID-19 Pandemic*, https://doi.org/10.1007/978-3-031-30844-4_5

107

burdens the health sector of countries far beyond what they can afford. The risk of a bottleneck in the healthcare system further increasing the mass mortality from this health disaster forces governments to implement immediate precautions against pandemics. On the other hand, these public health precautions directly change individuals' already established economic and societal relations. These mandatory changes in social life produce dissatisfaction among people.

Hence, the threat of transforming individual dissatisfaction into collective anger toward elected officials poses electoral risks. An increase in COVID-related death tolls or the danger of the collapse of health systems due to the excess demands creates pressure on political authorities to take immediate action. However, the danger of collective anger toward decision makers, which could result in election loss or mass protests or both, forces them to be more cautious due to the potential political cost of the restrictive public health measures.

Since the electoral return on implementing precautionary public health policies is ambiguous, politicians may fail to impose these restrictive measures at the socially optimal level. Comparative studies have revealed that federal democracies were more active than unitary democracies in combating the coronavirus (Shvetsova et al. 2021). However, the question remains as to what explains the differences among the decentralized systems in terms of which levels of government end up absorbing these political risks and enacting the politically costly public health measures.

Nigeria and South Africa are two primary examples of divergent task-sharing practices across levels of government in the fight against the COVID-19 pandemic. Figure 5.1 illustrates the difference between these two decentralized political systems. Nigerian federal incumbents mostly preferred to avoid the risk of appearing active in the policymaking process during the pandemic. In contrast, the central authorities in South Africa were the agents who took full responsibility for policies at both the regional and national levels.

Figure 5.1 plots the daily levels of a policy stringency index in order to capture incumbents' public health policy performance in Nigeria and South Africa in 2020. The Total Protective Policy Index (PPI) score is illustrated on the left-hand side. The Total PPI indicates the stringency of a country's public health pandemic policy from all combined measures implemented at all levels of government (Shvetsova et al. 2022). The index, as described in Chap. 1, is created by gathering data on national and subnational levels within eighteen public health categories, such as state of emergency, self-isolation, quarantine, border closures, and limits on social gatherings. Total PPI for the country is calculated as a weighted

5 CENTER-REGIONAL POLITICAL RISK SHARING IN THE COVID-19 PUBLIC...

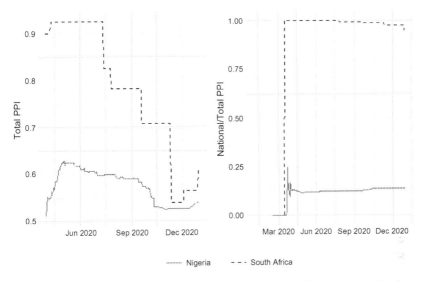

Fig. 5.1 Public health policy stringencies (left) and national governments' policy involvement (right) in Nigeria and South Africa. (Source: Shvetsova et al. 2022)

average of Total PPI of all regions in that country—an average of policy stringencies as observed in each region when both national and regional policies are considered. The illustration on the right indicates that the Total PPI score of South Africa, the dashed line, has a decreasing trend, and it reached almost the same level until late 2020 as the Total PPI of Nigeria, the red line.

In addition to Total PPI scores, the PPI dataset also calculates the index of policy responses of just the national policymakers, National PPI for a country on each day, as well as only Regional policymakers, Regional (for each region), and Average Regional (for the entire country) PPIs for each day (Shvetsova et al. 2022). Because the Total PPI for the country reflects the combined efforts of the two levels of government, using the ratio of National to Total PPIs captures the contribution of the central government in the fight against the pandemic.

The right panel of Fig. 5.1 shows a comparison of these relative contributions of the central governments in the public health policymaking process in the two countries. Notice how the Nigerian national government preferred to push risky policymaking onto the regions, whereas in South Africa the national government took over responsibility for policymaking almost entirely.

The difference in the level where government policies were produced in these two decentralized countries is striking. In what follows, I propose that the explanation of this difference lies in the differences in the way regional-national electoral processes in the two countries both connect and isolate regional electorates from the party elites at the two levels of government. I argue that the linkage among regional and national elites in the country's party system, the saliency of federal politics at the subnational level, and the federal constitutional design framing the nexus of regional- and national-level politics were three primary factors behind regional and national politicians' incentives to collaborate in public health policymaking during the pandemic.

Specifically, in Nigeria, weak party affiliations of regional elites with their parties and the lack of voters' attention to federal politics reduced the incentives for the federal government to protect their local counterparts from blame for implementing restrictive policies. The central government therefore contributed very little to the formulation of restrictive public health policies, and Nigerian national elites preferred instead to follow the credit-claiming strategy by leading in the distribution of in-kind and in-cash compensation to people dealing with the economic hardship of the pandemic. On the other hand, in South Africa, the constitutional design allows regional incumbents to link local issues with their regions' vote at the national level. Also, the strong party affiliation and the close party-list system raise the responsibilities of national political elites for their copartisan success in the regions and increase their incentives to enact restrictive public health policies that would apply in regions.

The rest of the chapter is organized as follows. Following an overview of politics and pandemic policies in Nigeria and South Africa (Section 5.2), Section 5.3 offers empirical support for my theoretical argument that the linkages among elites and between the voters and national incumbents have shaped national incumbents' making during the pandemic. Section 5.4 concludes the chapter.

5.2　Overview of Nigerian Politics and Its Impact on COVID-19 Policies

5.2.1　The Politics of Nigeria

After the military junta handed over the government peacefully in 1999, the Federal Republic of Nigeria consistently held elections at the national and state levels every four years. Regular elections have enabled Nigeria to progress toward successful democratization. Yet it is still characterized by a heavily regionalized party system, weak roots between society and parties, electoral violence, and an inadequacy of institutions for organizing elections, which render Nigerian democracy weak (Harry and Kalagbor 2021; Angerbrandt 2020).

From 1999 to 2015, the Peoples Democratic Party (PDP) was the only national party in Nigeria (Angerbrandt 2020). In 2013, six opposition parties built the All Progressive Congress (APC). After two years, the party competed nationwide and defeated the PDP in 2015 and 2019 in the presidential, national, and most local elections.

The weak national–regional party elite ties are an important factor in Nigerian politics. The disconnect in party organizations causes segregation between national and regional politicians. Elites use parties as a path to power and switch parties as a strategy for winning. Intraparty competition may be ruthlessly savage in regions where a party is strong because winning the party nomination also means securing a seat in parliament (Seeberg et al. 2018). Also, the weak ties between local and national political elites empower local strongmen who can directly impact state politics. Even in the two national parties, their electoral dominance hinges on patronage relations (Aniche et al. 2021).

Another peculiarity in Nigeria's political process is constituents' relative lack of interest in federal politics. This weakens parties' role in connecting national politicians with local-level incumbents. Citizens care more about state elections than national ballots, arguably because the platforms of national parties do not respond to local issues, and those are prioritized by the voters (Angerbrandt 2020). This disconnect is evidenced by the gap in the voter turnout rate in elections. Gubernatorial elections in thirty-six Nigerian states have on average 5 percent higher voter turnout than the presidential elections. This margin reaches as high as 20 percent for some states.

5.2.2 The Covid-19 Pandemic in Nigeria

From the first case recorded in mid-February to late December 2020, Nigeria Center for Disease Control (NCDC) reported more than 88,587 confirmed cases and 1289 COVID-related deaths (Dong et al. 2020). Whereas these case counts are relatively high compared to the rest of the world, the official numbers likely do not accurately reflect the magnitude

112 O. G. BAYRALI

Table 5.1 Snapshot of COVID-19 pandemic in some African countries

Country	Average daily cases per million	Average daily deaths per million	Average of daily tests per thousand	Estimated excess mortality rate per thousand	The ratio between the excess mortality rate and the reported Covid-19 mortality rate	Population
Botswana	20.65	0.06	0.22	399.50	7.03	2,588,423
Cameroon	3.21	0.06		70.30	22.32	27,198,628
Ethiopia	3.51	0.06	0.05	104.60	30.00	120,283,026
The Gambia	5.11	0.17		144.90	18.48	2,639,916
Ghana	5.69	0.04	0.07	58.30	27.75	32,833,031
Kenya	6.19	0.11	0.06	181.20	31.75	53,005,614
Mozambique	2.04	0.02	0.03	139.20	38.91	32,077,072
Namibia	32.29	0.46	0.37	395.60	4.95	2,530,151
Nigeria	**1.33**	**0.02**	**0.02**	**37.80**	**53.66**	213,401,323
Senegal	3.72	0.09	0.05	130.10	20.46	16,876,720
South Africa	**58.94**	**1.71**	**0.38**	**293.20**	**3.31**	59,392,255
Zimbabwe	3.03	0.08	0.06	283.60	16.16	15,993,524

Source: Wang et al. (2022); Hasell et al. (2020)

of the public health crisis in Nigeria due to the low testing rate (Campbell and McCaslin 2020). Table 5.1 compares the average daily cases and deaths per million and daily test rate per thousand for some African countries in 2020.

Compared to other African countries, Nigeria had dismal testing performance. The daily case and death rates that were reported were consequently extremely low. Table 5.1 also provides information about the excess mortality rate and the ratio between the excess mortality rate and the reported COVID-19 mortality rate. Nigeria had the lowest and highest ratios in these categories, respectively. In particular, the ratio between the excess mortality rate and the reported COVID-19 mortality rate may indicate that Nigerian authorities mostly underreported the public health cost of COVID-19.

Nigeria was equipped with clear federal-level institutional solutions for crisis management. The National Disaster Management Framework offers guidelines for intergovernmental cooperation to mitigate and recover from disasters (PreventionWeb 2010). Notably, if either the federal or state authorities shirk their responsibilities, this framework enables other agencies or level of government to take the initiative in each other's responsibilities (Abdulrauf 2021).

In addition to the Disaster Management Act, the prefederal Quarantine Act of 1926, which in fact was the basis of the 2020 Federal Covid-19 Regulations, allows the central government to encroach on the constitutional jurisdictions of state governments.

Despite these rights granted to the federal incumbent under the Disaster Management Act and the Quarantine Act, the biggest obstacle to the state-level fight against pandemics was the idleness of the federal government.[1] Regional incumbents had to act in areas of the federal government's responsibility, like closing land, sea, and air borders. For example, the states of Anambra, Bayelsa, Cross Rivers, Delta, and Imo announced the closure of federal roads and bridges (Aniche et al. 2021).

The entry of state governments into the constitutional realm of federal incumbents sparked political crises between federal and state governments. On April 7, 2020, the Rivers State government arrested two pilots and ten passengers for violating the air border closure. The Federal Aviation Minister accused the state government of not taking orders from the federal government, which is under the responsibility of federal authorities (Vanguard 2020).

The pandemic also hit the oil-dependent Nigerian economy. The International Monetary Fund (IMF) reported that the Nigerian economy experienced the worst recession in over 30 years due to the pandemic (The Cable 2020a). The central bank and federal government released recovery packages to compensate for the economic cost of the pandemic on small and medium-sized enterprises and economically disadvantaged groups. Tax relief, the reduction of crude oil prices, or interest rates are other components of the economic stimulus package that the federal authorities

---

[1] Even though President Buhari immediately launched a presidential task force to coordinate regional governments in the fight against the potential public health impact of COVID-19, the task force was dysfunctional (The Guardian 2020).

declared (KPMG 2020). Since the Nigerian economy is oil-dependent and more than 60% of the economy is informal, the federal government has limited fiscal power to soften the economic crisis. The European Union and IMF released emergent support to the government, around $3.5 billion in total, and provided some medical equipment (IMF 2020). The federal government was proactive in distributing this financial assistance without cooperation from regional authorities and claimed all credit for themselves.

Whereas the federal government launched an economic aid package, it abstained from imposing most of the public health restrictions. State governments had to bear the political costs of closing nonessential businesses, restaurants, or entertainment venues. Since federal resources were insufficient and allocated inefficiently, regional authorities could not compensate for the economic losses caused by these policies. As a result, state governments' stringent protective measures and limited resources led to social unrest in several cities.

Poor standards of care and the substandard diet of hospitalized COVID-19 patients and general hunger were prominent reasons for protests that erupted in Nigeria during the pandemic. During the protests, mostly the public facilities of regional authorities, specifically medical centers, were attacked and damaged (Sahara Reporters 2020).

Interestingly, the federal government did not respond to the pandemic-related content of the protests, even though it seemed sensitive to other protester demands. Thus, the federal government got involved in the political process of the dissolution of the Special Anti-Robbery Squad (SARS) as a result of an increase in the social unrest. Even though the inadequate government response to the pandemics also came to light during the demonstrations against corrupt security forces, the federal government again preferred to be a free rider, and most state governments made plans to defuse the social anger in this policy realm (VOA News 2020).[2]

---

[2] The biggest protest organized in late 2020 across the nation was the End SARS demonstrations. Despite the slogan, these demonstrations were unrelated to the pandemic. SARS referred to the Special Anti-Robbery Squad, an internal security unit created by the National Police Force in 1992 to fight robbery, kidnapping, and armed gangs. Over time this unit became the center of illegal activities, including illegal organ trade, rape, and home invasions (Al Jazeera 2020a). The nationwide protests organized in 2020 under the motto End SARS continued the previous year's string of demonstrations. The federal government disbanded this unit as the protests grew hard to control (The Cable 2020b).

5.3 SOUTH AFRICA

5.3.1 The Politics of South Africa

Post-apartheid political institutions in South Africa were intended to promote broad participation in which minority groups would be represented (Gouws and Mitchell 2005). Yet despite a proportional representation electoral system, which is believed to promote multipartyism, the South African party system is dominated by a single party headed by the African National Congress (ANC), with the so-called Tripartite Alliance consisting of the Congress of South African Trade Unions (Cosatu), the South African Communist Party, and the South African National Civic Organization as a minor coalition partner.

There are three tiers of government in South Africa. Since 1994, elections have been held once every five years for national, provincial, and municipal governments. The elections for the first two tiers are conducted concurrently, while the municipal elections lag by two years. The dominance of the ANC extends to the legislatures. The ANC is the governing party in eight out of nine provinces, with Western Cape as an exception.

Scholars explain the ANC single-party dominance by the distrust in the opposition parties because of their ties with the apartheid regime (Ferree 2010), although with new cohorts voting, this prejudice against the old parties is decreasing. Another reason ANC can safeguard its dominant power with consecutive electoral victories is its success in unifying anti-apartheid fractions (Booysen 2006).

The Democratic Alliance (DA) is the main opposition party; it received over 20 percent of the vote in the 2019 elections and has also been the center of both pre- and post-election alliances among the opposition parties. Pre-election alliances aim not at winning the national government but rather serving the desires of the leaders of the minor parties to secure a seat in parliament (Resnick 2013). However, in the Western Cape and some municipal governments, the partnerships led by the DA enabled opposition parties to win (Justesen and Schulz-Herzenberg 2018). Thus, with the rise of the DA, the South African party system may be transforming into an emerging two-party system with single-party dominance (Kotze and Bohler-Muller 2019). Furthermore, a new party, Economic Freedom Fighters (EFF), founded by politicians who left the ANC, entered the opposition on the left after the 2014 elections. After the 2019 general elections, the party increased its number of parliamentary seats from 25 to 45. Even though it is too early to predict whether the national party system will evolve from one of single-party dominance to a two-party or a multiparty system, these developments indicate that the ANC cannot take its dominance for granted and needs to actively maintain and expand its electoral linkages.

Close party-list proportional representation gives party leaders the key role in candidate selection and is one of the strongest influences empowering party leadership. This makes office seeking under the roof of a party a driving motivation for political elites. Not only does the close party-list system centralize the power within parties, but the additional unusual provision of dividing a single party list into equal-sized national and provincial lists gives party leaders direct control in regional elections and thus enhances the ties between a party's local and national political elites.

Another factor in forging ties between party incumbents and different levels of government is the selection rules to the national Senate. Senators are not directly elected but are chosen from provincial legislatures formed based on provincial election results. Thus, the Senate is de facto elected in provincial elections. Ten delegates from each province are permanent delegates appointed by the provincial legislatures based on the election. Four more delegates are the premier of the province and the three other delegates selected by the provincial legislature. Finally, six special delegates are rotated based on the subject discussed in the Senate. In this way, local political issues are nationalized, and the rotation helps every ward attain representation in the upper chamber.

Lastly, the ban on party switching or cross voting and the state funding of the parties proportionally to their electoral success are other regulatory mechanisms that improve the linkages among the partisan incumbents at all levels. Specifically, the act prohibiting floor crossing enables parties to empower intraparty discipline. The floor-crossing law at all levels of government requires MPs to give up their seats if they deviate from their party decisions (Hoeane 2008). This law increases the power of the party leadership and enables the incumbent party to increase its control over the governance of provinces and wards. The Public Funding Act increases the competitive power of national parties, especially the ANC, in elections at all levels and reduces the incentives for intraparty factional splits.

Finally, the consecutive election victories of the ANC at every tier of government have enabled the party elites to use the fiscal power of the central government as a reward/punishment mechanism (Ndletyana 2015). Fiscal resources are canalized to regional political actors depending on their loyalty. Such tactical redistribution of national resources increases the dependence of local political actors on national elites and links together their political futures, making national incumbents accountable for local outcomes.

5.3.2 *The Covid-19 Pandemic in South Africa*

On March 11, 2020, the WHO declared COVID-19 a pandemic. As cases worldwide rose, the South African national government was one of the fastest governments to respond to the crisis with drastic public health measures. On March 15, 2020, the president announced that the government had declared a national state of disaster.

As reported in Table 5.1, South Africa had the highest average daily testing rates among African countries. They also had the highest rates of COVID-19 infections and pandemic-related deaths. Compared to other African countries, South Africa had the lowest ratio of excess mortality to reported COVID-19 mortality. This ratio suggests minimal incentives for South African incumbents to conceal the true health costs of the pandemic.

The pandemic management in South Africa was centralized de facto, even though most responsibilities for the strategic planning of health services did not fall within the purview of the central government prior to the pandemic. The design of the healthcare system and the disaster management plan do not grant the center full authority but instead call for strong intergovernmental cooperation and coordination. The Disaster Management Act (2002) is the primary framework that establishes intergovernmental responsibilities as explicitly divided between national, provincial, and local governments. Provincial and local governments did not bear an equal burden in the pandemic decision-making, as mandated by this framework, but rather the burden was borne mostly by the national political incumbent (Steytler et al. 2021).

President Ramaphosa's government declared that its primary purpose was to organize the healthcare system against excessive demand that may emerge depending on the spread rate of the virus (Harris 2021). To this end, the government, in line with the recommendations of the National Coronavirus Command Council, officially declared a national state of disaster. President Ramaphosa introduced school closures and domestic travel restrictions on March 18, 2020, and a national lockdown on March 27, 2020, 22 days after the first detected case.

118   O. G. BAYRALI

Thus, the national policy response was dynamic and proportional to the pandemic ups and downs. The only strict lockdown was in the first period of the pandemic. After that, as new variants emerged, the restrictions went up but were kept in place for as short a time as possible.

The national government was also proactive in enacting economic policies to ease pandemic-related hardships. The virus arrived as a technical recession and stubborn unemployment was befalling the South African economy. Ramaphosa's administration revised the value-added tax rates for certain goods and released unemployment benefits and tax relief for businesses and individuals. The most striking of these fiscal supports was the R500 billion stimulus package announced as early as April 21, 2020. This package amounted to around 10 percent of South African GDP and was the heftiest one-time fiscal outlay, ten times bigger than the cost of hosting the World Cup 2010. Compared to international examples, the government's disbursement strategy was the most generous among emerging economies and higher than that of some advanced economies, such as South Korea and Canada (de Villiers et al. 2020).

The biggest obstacle to effective implementation of the public health policies was the mismanagement of resources to fight the pandemic. High-ranking politicians were involved in corruption scandals as they attempted to profit from allocating stimulus package funds, IMF funds, and irregular tenders for personal protection equipment (PPE) (Reuters 2020a). Thus President Ramaphosa's chief spokesperson, Khusela Diko, was accused of using her political connections to supply PPEs from her husband's firm (News 24 2020a). Similarly, the Education Department of the Gauteng Region embarrassed the central government with a corrupt tender to supply sanitization materials to schools (Parliamentary Monitoring Group 2020). The military and the Kwazulu-Natal government were similarly accused of making improper tenders (M & G 2020). The combination of the immense fiscal expansion, pandemic-damaged economy, and mismanagement of resources by public officials all created a need to borrow from the IMF for the first time in the post-apartheid period (The Economist 2020).

Another controversial issue that put the government in a politically tricky position was a concern over the potential erosion of civil liberties due to the intensity and length of the situation. After consecutive corruption scandals, civil society organizations and political parties again increased their pressure on Ramaphosa's administration. The DA used military force to inspect the lockdowns and curfews and filed a case against the National

5 CENTER-REGIONAL POLITICAL RISK SHARING IN THE COVID-19 PUBLIC... 119

Disaster Management Act, claiming that this act was enacted by bypassing parliamentary oversight. The Freedom Front Plus filed a court challenge over the same act regarding its constitutional validity (The South African Parliament Press Release 2020).

Hardship due to the stringent COVID-19 measures and the fallout from the corruption scandals increased the pressure on the government. The opposition parties organized several protests across provinces to pressure the government politically. They also applied to regional courts to repeal some of the COVID-19 regulations (Reuters 2020b). [3]

The protests in the early period of the lockdown were generally about the inefficient allocation of food parcels, poverty, or the lack of clean water in some regions (Open Democracy 2020). After the corruption scandals, the pace of demonstrations accelerated. People directed their anger at corrupt public authorities and the mismanagement of resources, including health workers, taxi drivers, service-sector workers, and restaurant and hotel owners (Al Jazeera 2020b). In several cities around the country, people organized protests regarding governments' inadequate compensation for the economic cost of the pandemic.

Government's response to these protests was sometimes repressive. Police forces used tear gas or water cannons in some Johannesburg and Cape Town demonstrations (Taiwan News 2020). However, the protests forced the government to scale back its COVID-19 policies to below optimal levels. The The Ramaphosa administration also enacted the Infection Prevention and Control (IPC) law to improve working conditions for healthcare workers (WHO 2020). In the transportation sector as well, new regulations were implemented to increase passenger capacities (The South African Government Press Release 2020). Finally, due to accusations of corruption, the president's chief spokesperson and the Gauteng Provincial Health Minister were forced to step down. A group of auditors was authorized to independently investigate all corruption cases (WSWS 2020).

---

[3] The tobacco ban was one of the hot topics on which opposition parties admonished the government harshly. Even though the Ramaphosa government insisted on enforcing the ban, after the Democratic Alliance's (DA) continuous effort beginning in late May, the Western Cape High Court repealed the ban by finding this regulation unconstitutional (News 24 2020b).

5.4 Discussion and Concluding Remarks

This chapter scrutinized how party affiliation among elites affected intergovernmental task sharing during the pandemic in two decentralized African countries, Nigeria and South Africa. While the pandemic management process was almost entirely the responsibility of the central government in South Africa, the process was carried out by state governments due to the idleness of the federal government in Nigeria. Based on the narrative built in the preceding sections, this analysis argued that the remarkable divergence of the intergovernmental task sharing in these countries during the pandemics hinged on whether parties could facilitate strong intraparty linkages between federal and regional elites as well as between voters and elites.

In Nigeria, elites utilize political parties as a means to bolster their positions at the local level. Local strongmen switch their parties repeatedly to enlarge their power base in their regions. Voters are primarily loyal to individuals rather than to parties, and they are politically mobile as the elites they support change their party.

Another linkage problem in Nigerian politics is between the society and the federal elites. The saliency of federal politics at the regional level is low, reducing electoral pressure on federal elites. Hence, staying away from the regional-level policymaking process is a more profitable strategy for federal elites.

Finally, the constitutional design of Nigerian federalism cannot establish a vital link between federal and regional politics. The Senate is organized as a legislative body to produce national-level policies. Directly elected members from each state in national elections have no legal responsibilities to bridge the gap between regional and national politics.

Weak ties among elites and the low importance of federal politics at the local level caused a cooperation problem in fighting the pandemic, summing up well why the federal government failed to fulfill its constitutional responsibilities in combating the pandemic in Nigeria. This idleness forced state governments to overstep their constitutional power, whereas the limited fiscal capacity of the state governments created inefficiencies and public dissatisfaction.

In South Africa, political parties are the primary policy actors. The rigid constraints that hamper party switching strengthen intraparty discipline. The financial limits on newly established parties shrink their power during political campaigns compared to established parties. These regulations reduce the risk of divergence of intraparty elites' electoral incentives.

Also, the close party-list system enhances the role of the national party elites in the party organization. Even though provincial quotas present local politicians with opportunities to be active in national politics, the likelihood that regional politicians will properly represent their constituencies does not diminish the solid intraparty authority of the national elites.

Even though party organization is centralized in South Africa, South African politics allows regional politicians to have a voice at the national level compared to Nigeria. The organization of the Senate enables premiers and politicians from provincial parliaments to bring local political issues to the national political playing field. Thus, local political issues directly impact the interparty political struggle at the federal level.

In the story of the South African COVID-19 experience, the reason an almost centralized policy path was taken was because the centralized party organizations enjoyed relatively strong linkages between provincial and national elites. In other words, the stringent policies, which were harsh enough to spark protests and therefore carried political risks, showed that the risk appetite of the central government was high due to the possible political costs. One of the most fundamental of these political risks was the incompetence of provincial governments in the fight against the pandemic, which threatened the political future of national actors. Therefore, the federal government intervened directly in cases where provincial executive bodies were not up to the task of dealing with the pandemic.

As a final remark, this research did not treat the South African party system as a notable example of how political authorities should respond to an exogenous shock in a decentralized system. Instead, the analysis presented here aimed to discuss the negative impact of the imbalanced linkage among elites in connection with implementing policies across jurisdictions. Additionally, the reduced importance of national politics does not mean that regional party systems produce collective goods less efficiently and below the socially optimal level, as in the case of Nigeria. Fiscally empowered local authorities with strong electoral accountability may also push decision makers to produce local collective goods optimally.

References

Abdulrauf L (2021) Managing Covid-19 in a 'Façade Federalism': The case of Nigeria. In: Steytler N (ed) Comparative Federalism and Covid-19. Routledge, New York, p 355–372.

Al Jazeera (2020a) Nigeria's SARS: A brief history of the Special Anti-Robbery Squad. https://www.aljazeera.com/features/2020/10/22/sars-a-brief-history-of-a-rogue-unit. Accessed 24 Sep 2022.

Al Jazeera (2020b) South Africa healthcare workers protest, threaten strike. https://www.aljazeera.com/news/2020/9/3/south-africa-healthcare-workers-protest-threaten-strike. Accessed 6 Oct 2022.

Angerbrandt H (2020) Party system institutionalization and the 2019 state elections in Nigeria. Regional & Federal Studies 30(3):415–440.

Aniche ET, Iwuoha VC, Obi KC (2021) Covid-19 containment policies in Nigeria: the role of conflictual federal–state relations in the fight against the pandemic. Review of African Political Economy 48(169):442–451.

Booysen S (2006) The will of the parties versus the will of the people? Defections, elections and alliances in South Africa. Party Politics 12(6):727–746.

Campbell J, McCaslin J (2020) How Nigeria Has Responded to Covid-19 So Far. Available via https://www.cfr.org/blog/how-nigeria-has-responded-covid-19-so-far. Accessed 16 Nov 2022.

de Villiers C, Cerbone D, Van Zijl W (2020) The South African government's response to Covid-19. Journal of Public Budgeting, Accounting & Financial Management.

Dong, E, Du H, Gardner L (2020) An interactive web-based dashboard to track COVID-19 in real time. The Lancet infectious diseases 20(5): 533–534.

Hasell J, Mathieu E, Beltekian D, Macdonald B, Giattino C, Ortiz-Ospina E, Ritchie H (2020) A cross-country database of COVID-19 testing. Scientific data 7(1):1–7.

Gouws A, Mitchell P (2005) South Africa: one party dominance despite perfect proportionality. The Politics of Electoral Systems 353–374.

Ferree KE (2010) Framing the race in South Africa: The political origins of racial census elections. Cambridge University Press.

Harris J (2021) The politics of coronavirus response in south Africa. Coronavirus Politics: The Comparative Politics and Policy of COVID-19.

Harry D, Kalagbor SB (2021) Electoral Violence and Democratic Consolidation in Nigeria: Issues and Challenges. Advances in Social Sciences Research Journal 8(7).

Hoeane T (2008) Floor-crossing in South Africa: entrenching or undermining democracy?. Politeia 27(2):70–88.

IMF (2020) IMF Executive Board approves US$ 3.4 billion in emergency support to Nigeria to address the COVID-19 pandemic. Press Release No:20/191.

https://www.imf.org/en/News/Articles/2020/04/28/pr20191-nigeria-imf-executive-board-approves-emergency-support-to-address-covid-19. Accessed 24 Sep 2022.

Justesen MK, Schulz-Herzenberg C (2018) The decline of the African national congress in South Africa's 2016 municipal elections. Journal of Southern African Studies 44(6):1133–1151.

Kotze JS, Bohler-Muller N (2019) Quo Vadis? Reflections on the 2019 South African General Elections. Politikon 46(4):365–370.

KPMG (2020) Nigeria: Government and institution measures in response to COVID-19. https://home.kpmg/xx/en/home/insights/2020/04/nigeria-government-and-institution-measures-in-response-to-covid.html. Accessed 8 July 2022.

M & G (2020) Blanket scandal exposes potential for Covid-19 corruption. https://mg.co.za/article/2020-04-16-blanket-scandal-exposes-potential-for-covid-19-corruption/. Accessed 11 Oct 2022.

Ndletyana M (2015) African national Congress: From an emancipatory to a rent-seeking instrument. Transformation: Critical Perspectives on Southern Africa 87(1): 95–116.

News 24 (2020a) President's spokesperson Khusela Diko takes leave of absence in face of PPE procurement scandal. https://www.news24.com/news24/south-africa/news/presidents-spokesperson-khusela-diko-takes-leave-of-absence-in-face-of-ppe-procurement-scandal-20200727. Accessed 5 Oct 2022.

News 24 (2020b) Western Cape High Court rules that lockdown regulations are justified, dismisses application. https://www.news24.com/news24/south-africa/news/western-cape-high-court-rules-that-lockdown-regulations-are-justified-dismisses-application-20200626. Accessed 6 Oct 2022.

Open Democracy (2020) "We are still waiting" – protesting under lockdown in South Africa. https://www.opendemocracy.net/en/beyond-trafficking-and-slavery/we-are-still-waiting-protesting-under-lockdown-in-south-africa/. Accessed 5 Oct 2022.

Parliamentary Monitoring Group (2020) Gauteng Provincial Government on its COVID-19 response plans. https://pmg.org.za/page/GautengProvincialGovernmentonitsCOVID19responseplans. Accessed 8 Oct 2022.

PreventionWeb (2010) Nigeria: National disaster framework. https://www.preventionweb.net/publication/nigeria-national-disaster-framework. Accessed 16 Nov 2022.

Resnick D (2013) Do electoral coalitions facilitate democratic consolidation in Africa?. Party Politics 19(5):735–757.

Reuters (2020a) South African corruption watchdog probes Covid-19 tenders. https://www.reuters.com/article/us-health-coronavirus-safrica-corruption-idUSKCN24Z2EU. Accessed 5 Oct 2022.

124 O. G. BAYRALI

Reuters (2020b) Court rules some South African lockdown restrictions invalid. https://www.reuters.com/article/us-health-coronavirus-safrica-court-idUSKBN2392BV. Accessed 6 Oct 2022.

Sahara Reporters (2020) Covid-19 patients protest, threaten to abscond over poor treatment in Niger State. https://saharareporters.com/2020/05/06/covid-19-patients-protestthreaten-abscond-over-poor-treatment-niger-state. Accessed 8 July 2022.

Seeberg MB, Wahman M, Skaaning SE (2018). Candidate nomination, intra-party democracy, and election violence in Africa. Democratization 25(6):959–977.

Shvetsova O, VanDusky-Allen J, Zhirnov A, Adeel A B, Catalano, Catalano O, ... Zhao T (2021) Federal institutions and strategic policy responses to COVID-19 pandemic. Frontiers in Political Science, 3(66).

Shvetsova O et al (2022) Protective Policy Index (PPI) global dataset of origins and stringency of COVID 19 mitigation policies. Scientific data 9(1): 1–10.

Steytler N, de Visser J, Chigwata T (2021) South Africa: Surfing towards centralisation on the Covid-19 wave. In: Steytler N (ed) Comparative Federalism and Covid-19. Routledge, New York, p 336–354.

Taiwan News (2020) South African police disperse protestors over lockdown pain. https://www.taiwannews.com.tw/en/news/3973613. Accessed 7 Oct 2022.

The Cable (2020a) Travel ban, lockdown, protest... how COVID-19, #EndSARS shaped 2020. https://www.thecable.ng/travel-ban-lockdown-protest-how-covid-19-endsars-shaped-2020. Accessed 8 July 2022.

The Cable (2020b) IMF: Nigeria heading into its worst recession in over 30 years. https://www.thecable.ng/breaking-nigeria-heading-into-its-worst-recession-in-30-years-says-imf. Accessed 8 July 2022.

The Economist (2020) South Africa borrows from the IMF for the first time since apartheid. https://www.economist.com/middle-east-and-africa/2020/07/30/south-africa-borrows-from-the-imf-for-the-first-time-since-apartheid. Accessed 5 Oct 2022.

The Guardian (2020) Buhari names task force on coronavirus. https://guardian.ng/news/buhari-names-task-force-on-coronavirus/. Accessed 8 July 2022.

The South African Government Press Release (2020) Transport on revised directions regulating public transport operations during Coronavirus COVID-19 lockdown period. https://www.gov.za/speeches/transport-revised-directions-regulating-public-transport-operations-during-coronavirus. Accessed 7 Oct 2022.

The South African Parliament Press Release (2020) Dismissal of Freedom Front Plus Disaster Management Act Court Challenge. https://www.parliament.gov.za/press-releases/dismissal-freedom-front-plus-disaster-management-act-court-challenge. Accessed 6 Oct 2022.

5 CENTER-REGIONAL POLITICAL RISK SHARING IN THE COVID-19 PUBLIC... 125

Vanguard News (2020) Exxon Mobil staff: I won't take orders from Abuja-Wike. https://www.vanguardngr.com/2020/04/exxonmobil-staff-i-wont-takeorders-from-abuja-wike/. Accessed 8 July 2022.

Voa News (2020) Nigerians justify massive looting of COVID-19 supplies. https://www.voanews.com/a/covid-19-pandemic_nigerians-justify-massive-looting-covid-19-supplies/6197611.html. Accessed 8 July 2022.

Wang H, Paulson KR, Pease SA, Watson S, Comfort H, Zheng P, Murray CJ (2022) Estimating excess mortality due to the COVID-19 pandemic: a systematic analysis of COVID-19-related mortality, 2020–21. The Lancet 399(10334):1513–1536

WHO (2020) South Africa steps up hygiene in health facilities to protect against COVID-19. https://www.who.int/news-room/feature-stories/detail/south-africa-steps-up-hygiene-in-health-facilities-to-protect-against-covid-19. Accessed 7 Oct 2022.

WSWS (2020) South African health care workers strike as opposition to ANC government mounts. https://www.wsws.org/en/articles/2020/09/09/safr-s09.html. Accessed 7 Oct 2022.

CHAPTER 6

Pick Your Poison: Political Expediencies, Economic Necessities, and COVID-19 Response in Malaysia and Indonesia

Tian Yi Zhao

6.1 INTRODUCTION

As neighboring countries in Southeast Asia, Malaysia and Indonesia share many geographical and social characteristics. Both reside on the same archipelago, have similar demographics and religions, command fast-growing economies, and are considered fledgling democracies. When the COVID-19 virus spread to the region in 2020, it struck the two countries in roughly equal scope and severity, causing public health crises throughout (Amul et al. 2022). The contagious and lethal nature of the COVID-19 pandemic warranted a rapid response in both countries. Surprisingly, the Malaysian government and the Indonesian government implemented rather dissimilar response policies. Conventional political beliefs may attribute the difference to government structures or partisan dispositions, as

---

T. Zhao (✉)
Department of Political Science, Binghamton University, Binghamton, NY, USA
e-mail: tzhao19@binghamton.edu

© The Author(s), under exclusive license to Springer Nature Switzerland AG 2023
O. Shvetsova (ed.), *Government Responses to the COVID-19 Pandemic*, https://doi.org/10.1007/978-3-031-30844-4_6

127

the Malaysian government is federal and more right-leaning, while the Indonesian government is unitary and more left-leaning (Toshkov et al. 2021). Next they would predict that the Indonesian government would implement more stringent policy measures than its Malaysian counterpart, since unitary structure and left-wing positions are usually associated with government intervention and centralization. But in reality, it was the Malaysian government that implemented more stringent policy measures, to the degree that they even raised democratic and human rights concerns (Hashim et al. 2021; Djalante et al. 2020). Hence, the difference in the COVID-19 policy responses between Malaysia and Indonesia constitutes an important puzzle: why would a right-leaning, federal government implement more stringent policy measures than a left-leaning, unitary one?

Instead of political structures, I argue in this study that COVID-19 response policies in Malaysia and Indonesia were determined by political expediencies and economic necessities, factors that are both contingent and contextual. It should be noted that these factors are *not* meant to be mutually exclusive—after all, economic considerations often enter into political calculations, just as political choices may very well impact economic performances. For the purposes of this study, however, political expediencies are used to denote solely direct power calculations about how to hold onto office and/or maintain legislative majorities. Economic necessities, on the other hand, reflect only the economic cost of implementing policies, in this case response measures to fight the spread of COVID-19. The policy choices by the Malaysian and Indonesian governments are then understood as the products of these factors: each leadership determined the level of policy stringency in accordance with its political incentives and economic opportunities of action. Only when stringent policy measures can serve certain political purposes and actually be afforded are such measures chosen.

From this perspective, the Malaysian government was mired in political crisis and faced continuous challenges to its rule, but it was also better endowed economically and technologically to absorb the cost of varying policy measures against COVID-19. Hence, it was incentivized to suspend the political process by implementing stringent policy measures that would keep opponents and voters at home. Government closures and traveling restrictions were questionable but legitimate means to expand power and extend survival. In comparison, the Indonesian government was in a more stable political position, with its president enjoying strong majority support without threats of legislative coup or reelection. This

6 PICK YOUR POISON: POLITICAL EXPEDIENCIES, ECONOMIC NECESSITIES... 129

means it was less incentivized to implement stringent policy measures. But Indonesia's backward economic conditions also restricted its set of choices. If the Indonesian government had decided to implement stringent policy measures, then the economic cost could have been exceedingly high, as its economy is not well structured to withstand lockdowns, closures, and other restrictions. In summary, the levels of policy stringency in Malaysia and Indonesia are determined in part by political expediencies and economic necessities. When there are political incentives to implement stringent policy measures *and* economic capacities to bear the cost, then such measures are chosen. This should happen in Malaysia, but not in Indonesia.

One of the main objectives of this study, therefore, is to introduce a theoretical framework for understanding the contingent nature of policy choices, especially during times of great uncertainty and instability. The COVID-19 pandemic is a global, catastrophic event; it has challenged modern life and governance in ways unlike any previous events. Similarly, the pandemic has also contested the explanatory power of our theories and the centralities of the associated political concepts and methods. Could policy choices be adequately explained in terms of political structures, partisan dispositions, and/or regime types? If those systemic influences do not offer a sufficient explanation, then what other factors should we consider? And how do we assess them among the constellation of social forces and individual action? In this study, I will test a theoretical framework of short-term contextual strategic influences by examining the policy choices of the Malaysian and the Indonesian governments in response to the COVID-19 pandemic. The next section analyzes Malaysia's and Indonesia's short-term strategic environments as shaped by their political and economic conditions at the time of the pandemic onset. Section 6.3 discusses incumbents' policy choices in the context and contingent on their short-term incentive structures. The final section presents conclusions.

6.2 POLITICAL AND ECONOMIC CONDITIONS IN MALAYSIA

At the start of the COVID-19 pandemic, Malaysia's political context, beyond institutional influences, encompassed incumbents' in-the-moment challenges and calculations as well as its structural, economic endowment, which could have constrained policy implementations. Specifically, the ruling coalition was in the midst of a political crisis and has just recently narrowly prevailed over the opposition. Meanwhile, the country was more economically and technologically endowed than most of its neighbors, and especially Indonesia. As a result, the Malaysian government was politically incentivized to use stringent COVID-19 response measures, because in addition to their public health value, they had the side effect of suppressing the opposition and, thus, neutralizing the most immediate political threat to the incumbent. On top of the public health restrictions, the government declared a national state of emergency and suspended both legislative and electoral processes, thereby blocking all channels for oppositional action. Malaysian national incumbents' policy choices in response to the pandemic were consistent with the short-term incentives that emerged in the political context. The economic endowment did not constrain the government's response because of the characteristics of the labor force.

6.2.1 Malaysia's Cabinet Fragility

The still ongoing political crisis in Malaysia started when its former prime minister, Mahathir Mohamad, refused to hand over power to his designated successor, Anwar Ibrahim. Mahathir and Anwar were once fierce political rivals but partnered in an unlikely alliance to win the 2018 general election, defeating the right-wing coalition that had ruled Malaysia since its independence in 1957. In early 2020, Mahathir's supporters attempted to form a new coalition in order to extend his reign and prevent Anwar from assuming office as promised. The breakdown of the agreement caused a rift within the ruling Pakatan Harapan (PH) coalition, as dozens of Parliament members decided to withdraw their support, led by Muhyiddin Yassin's Malaysian United Indigenous Party (BERSATU). In a move known as the Sheraton coup, Muhyiddin formed an alliance with parties that lost the 2018 election, namely, the United Malays National Organization Party (UMNO), the Pan-Malaysian Islamic Party (PAS), and the Sarawak Parties Alliance (GPS). When Mahathir became aware of the plan, especially BERSATU's alliance with UMNO, he abruptly resigned his position as prime minister, thereby ending the government and plunging the country into political crisis.

Facing sudden and unexpected political instability, the king of Malaysia, Al-Sultan Abdullah, met with every member of Parliament in March 2020 to determine which leader could command majority support and ultimately named Muhyiddin as the new prime minister. The legitimacy of Muhyiddin's cabinet, however, continued to be questioned. Opponents and political observers argued that Muhyiddin did not win the office through democratic means. At the same time, Muhyiddin's coalition had only a slim majority, with 114 out of 222 seats in Parliament. This empowered his key allies in the coalition who often threatened to withdraw support, which would mean the collapse of the government and the removal of Muhyiddin as prime minister. Muhyiddin's government therefore was experiencing a serious legitimacy crisis.

With the government thus mired in a political crisis, Muhyiddin had strong incentives for implementing some drastic policies that would suppress the opposition and solidify his power. To be fair, he did try alternative political strategies, for example, attempting to obtain ten additional legislative seats, such as when he pushed for the demise of the Sabah state government to pressure its chief minister, Shafie Apdal. That move failed, and Shafie responded by dissolving his state assembly in July 2020. The subsequent state election in September 2020 not only caused COVID-19 cases to spike but also led to a clash within Muhyiddin's already weakened coalition. Although BERSATU and UMNO did align to form a new state government after competing in the Sabah election, leaders of UMNO had become increasingly frustrated by the coalition, as they felt that Muhyiddin held power only thanks to a slim majority and that their support was not sufficiently appreciated. Some of them joined Muhyiddin's so-called Sheraton coup in exchange for an evasion of corruption charges, but the promise was not kept once the new government was formed. Feeling alienated, they planned to form an alliance with Anwar for another parliamentary coup to overthrow Muhyiddin. Anwar stated on September 23 that he had secured a "strong, formidable and convincing" majority in Parliament.

Hence, Muhyiddin was in a perilous position. He could have followed the conventional procedure and called a general election immediately, but it would have been one that he was unlikely to win. The drastic rise of COVID-19 cases in Sabah offered him another option, albeit an unusual and unconventional one. His government could implement stringent policy measures and keep both his opponents and voters at home, all while containing the spread of the virus, which would be a righteous cause. This could be achieved by declaring a national state of emergency and enacting a comprehensive policy program that would close public offices and restrict social activities and mass travel. This would allow the government to suspend legislative and electoral processes at least temporarily and

132   T. ZHAO

preempt its political opponents from challenging the government, without openly violating democratic precepts and coming into conflict with the constitutional framework.

6.2.2   Binding Economic Constraints on Policy Adoption

The use of stringent policy measures against the pandemic, however, could be constrained by an economy that is unable to absorb their associated costs. Significant economic capacity on the part of both the government and the workforce is required to bear the costs of lockdowns, closures, and various other restrictions. Without adequate resources and resilience, stringent pandemic policies could create a net political loss for the government due to the overwhelming burden on the population and the resulting unrest. Fortunately, Malaysia was reasonably well endowed economically and technologically in terms of absorbing the costs of the stringent public health policies. Malaysia's comparative advantages enabled its economy and workforce to withstand the negative impacts of the drastic policy measures, and this expanded the range of feasible policy strategies for the Muhyiddin government. This is evidenced by an assessment of Malaysia's economic conditions after a set of strict policy measures known as the Movement Control Order (MCO) was implemented: it was centralized, comprehensive, and stringent, but not economically crippling (Hashim et al. 2021).

When the MCO was implemented from early 2020 to late 2021, most workers in Malaysia adjusted relatively well, at least in comparison to workers in neighboring Southeast Asian countries (Djalante et al. 2020). About 44% of workers surveyed by the Malaysian government reported that they were working from home, as nonessential businesses and services were forced to close. Further, 16.2% faced shorter working hours, about the same number of workers lost their jobs, while 10.9% of workers were put on leave without pay; 7.4% of the workforce was largely unaffected (Malaysia Department of Statistics 2020). Rahman et al. (2020) found that around 35% of jobs in Malaysia could plausibly be performed at home. The statistics are lower than those in the United States but higher than in the European Union (37% and 17%, respectively) (Dingel and Neiman 2020). Taken together, it appears that most Malaysian workers could bear the costs of lockdowns and other stringent policy measures. There were certainly inequalities among workers, but in general they fared well—better than the Indonesian workforce, which will be discussed in the next section (Khatiwada et al. 2021).

One of Malaysia's comparative advantages lies in its technological and infrastructural support (Ling et al. 2021). The capacity to work from home depends on whether workers have necessary hardware, such as computers and Internet connectivity at home. Recent data from Malaysia's Department of Statistics show that 71.3% of households have computers, and 90.1% have an Internet connection. Furthermore, workers in the finance, real estate, and information and communication technology (ICT) sectors have 100% computer and Internet access, as these sectors also engage in high-return economic activities (Rahman et al. 2020). To help workers transition to their new work settings, the Malaysian government offered tax relief for purchases of electronic devices that were conducive to work-from-home arrangements. But even before the pandemic, the Malaysian government had already been trying to spur technological advancements and, more specifically, Industrial Revolution 4.0, an initiative that aimed to infuse automation into various sectors of the Malaysian economy. These factors enabled the Malaysian workforce to better absorb the cost of implementing stringent policy measures against COVID-19. In other words, the Muhyiddin government had fewer economic constraints when choosing its pandemic policies.

6.3   MALAYSIA'S COVID-19 RESPONSE

With both political incentives and economic capacities in place, Muhyiddin indeed chose the more stringent policy options (Fauzi and Paiman 2021). The most politically impactful and controversial policy was the national state of emergency declared from January 2021 to August 2021. During the initial stages of the COVID-19 pandemic, the Malaysian government was mostly able to keep the spread of the virus under control. But the snap election held at Sabah in September 2020—as a result of Muhyiddin's political maneuvers—contributed to the third wave of COVID-19 infections. Case numbers quickly climbed, primarily in the states of Sabah and Kedah. Malaysia's total cases were approaching 100,000.

Malaysia's public health conditions were bleak, but the political opportunities for action were ripe. Before the parliamentary session in November 2020, Muhyiddin promptly asked the king of Malaysia to declare a national state of emergency, but the king rejected the proposal after consulting with other heritage rulers. This did not deter Muhyiddin, as he prepared for another attempt and turned down opportunities to negotiate with UMNO and opposition members. Political infighting soon broke out. In

December 2020, UMNO and other parties aligned to defeat BERSATU in Perak's state assembly, further weakening Muhyiddin's coalition. When Parliament voted for the new budget in late December, the governing coalition received only 111 votes, while the opposition received 108. Some UMNO members were also beginning to withdraw their support for Muhyiddin, including former minister Nazri Aziz.

By all accounts, Muhyiddin then was a politically weak prime minister on the verge of losing power and even office, until the COVID-19 pandemic provided him with a unique opportunity to ensure his political survival. If Muhyiddin could shut down legislative and electoral processes, especially for somewhat legitimate purposes, then he would be able to rule without formal oversight and challenges. Such power would be controversial but unfettered. This gave Muhyiddin strong political incentives to keep trying drastic strategies.

At the turn of the year, Muhyiddin asked the nation's monarch again to declare a national state of emergency. This time the king finally agreed and declared a national emergency on January 12, 2021. It suspended all parliamentary activities, thereby enabling the government to introduce laws without oversight and approval and preventing legislators from forming new coalitions. The emergency declaration also paused federal, regional, and local elections, so that Muhyiddin's coalition would not be challenged at the polls (Amul et al. 2022). It was set to be effective until August 1, 2021, conditional on the severity of the pandemic. At the same time, the federal government also imposed lockdowns in major cities such as Kuala Lumpur, banning international travel and a variety of social activities. Nonessential businesses and services were closed, as was Parliament and certain government offices (Arnakim and Kibtiah 2021). This was the first *national* emergency the Malaysian government had declared since 1969, when Parliament was suspended after racial riots broke out between ethnic Malays and Chinese in Kuala Lumpur. The riots caused almost 200 deaths and delayed legislative activities until 1971. A half century later, the Malaysian government would declare a national state of emergency again, this time the rationale on paper was the drastic rise in COVID-19 infections and deaths.

Opponents and independent observers argued that the national emergency declaration was designed to allow Muhyiddin's precarious coalition to evade scrutiny and cling to power. It handed immense emergency powers to Muhyiddin and his government without effective legislative oversight. Many worried that the emergency declaration would undermine democracy in Malaysia and enable Muhyiddin to rule arbitrarily and continuously. According to Civicus, a nonprofit organization that focuses on citizen action and civil society, Malaysia's emergency declaration "seems like another attempt by Muhyiddin to hold on to power, block elections and to remove parliamentary oversight, rather than to seriously address the pandemic." Nik Ahmad Kamal Nik Mahmood, a professor at the International Islamic University of Malaysia, similarly asserted that the emergency declaration granted substantial emergency powers to the current government. "If Parliament is not in session," Mahmood told *The Guardian*, "the government has the power to make laws, the constitution is more or less suspended, as a substantial part of it can be overridden by emergency law" (Ratcliffe 2021). The move had thus cast an ominous shadow on Malaysia's democracy, reversing the gains from the 2018 election, when Mahathir and Anwar aligned to defeat the Barisan Nasional (BN) coalition.

Besides the national emergency declaration, Malaysia's national policy program was stringent and centralized (Fauzi and Paiman 2021). From March 2020 to November 2021, the Malaysian government implemented the MCO throughout the country. It included the prohibition of mass movement and social gatherings, restrictions on international and regional travel, and closures of schools, nonessential businesses, and certain government offices, among other stringent policy measures (Hashim et al. 2021). Those who violated the order could be subjected to fines, community service, jail time, and/or criminal prosecution. In April 2020, Minister of Defense Ismail Sabri Yaakob reported that 4,189 individuals had been arrested for violating the MCO, of whom 1,449 individuals had been charged in court. Jail sentences could range from two days to several months. Even when compared across the world, Malaysia's MCO was considered one of the most stringent policy programs. Moreover, the policy measures contained within the MCO were also implemented relatively consistently throughout the country. The Malaysian federal government took the initiative by itself rather than relying on regional and local governments for implementation and enforcement. Muhyiddin announced the order on March 16, 2020, and extended it numerous times. It was commonly called a "national lockdown" in public discourse, signifying the scope and stringency of its measures. Regional and local governments could adopt their own policies against COVID-19 as well, but only as supplements to the national policy program.

6.4 Political and Economic Conditions in Indonesia

In stark contrast, the Indonesian government's response to the COVID-19 pandemic was much less centralized and stringent (Arnakim and Kibtiah 2021). Although Indonesia shared many geographical and social characteristics with Malaysia, their respective political and economic conditions differed, and this became the basis of their different COVID-19 response. To begin with, the Indonesian government was in a much stronger political position than its counterpart in Malaysia. Its president, Joko "Jokowi" Widodo, was elected with a wide margin in the 2014 and the 2019 elections; he had no reelection concerns. His governing coalition also enjoyed an overwhelming majority in Parliament, with 471 out of 575 seats under its control in the lower house. There were no oppositional forces that could realistically challenge Jokowi's government; its political standing was almost as firm as it could possibly have been. Jokowi's personal popularity was also relatively high throughout the pandemic. Polls released by Lembaga Survei Indonesia in 2020 and 2021 showed that his approval rating hovered around 60%.

In dealing with the COVID-19 pandemic, the Indonesian government thus was not sufficiently incentivized to implement more stringent policy measures, at least from a political standpoint. The legislative and the electoral processes served the government well, so the government was not looking for an opportunity to interfere with either. President Jokowi was popular and powerful enough to govern as he wished. Unlike Muhyiddin in Malaysia, Jokowi needed political *normalcy* rather than its opposite. Stringent policy measures against COVID-19 would disturb that normalcy and bring instability to a much greater extent than in Malaysia, as millions of Indonesians would be forced to leave their workplace and urban areas for reasons that will be discussed in the next section.

Unlike in Malaysia, the Indonesian economy imposed binding constraints on the harshness of the public health measures the government could impose. Indonesia is one of the fastest growing countries in the world, yet it remains at a relatively low level of economic development. The structure of the economy and the condition of the labor force restricted the range of feasible policy choices for pandemic response, because the economy could not absorb the cost of stringent policy measures (Ling et al. 2021). Indonesia had around 70 million industrial workers, most in blue-collar manufacturing sectors, who would be profoundly impacted by stringent policy measures such as lockdowns, closures, and social and traveling restrictions. Micro, small, and medium-sized enterprises (MSMEs) had suffered the most economically as a result of the pandemic and associated response policies. These smaller enterprises—ranging from cigarette stands and hair salons to motorbike taxis and massage parlors—constituted the lifeline of Indonesia's economy and affected every aspect of social life. They employed the vast majority (97%) of Indonesia's 135 million workforce and had largely kept the economy afloat, even during previous financial crises (Atmojo and Fridayani 2021).

The Indonesian economy had suffered a significant setback as a result of the COVID-19 pandemic, even before stringent policy measures were implemented spatially and temporally (Djalante et al. 2020). It contracted for the first time since the Asian financial crisis of 1997–1998. According to the government, the COVID-19 pandemic had already caused millions of Indonesians to lose their jobs and/or fall below poverty lines (Khatiwada et al. 2021). Although the economy had rebounded in the second quarter of 2021, economic forecasts predicted that its growth rate was likely to decrease again, after the spread of the Delta variant and subsequent policy measures against those were put in place. As observed by Marcus Mietzner of Australian National University, "The country has now seen four successive quarters of economic contraction, and the current spike in cases will prolong the crisis" (Aditya and Heijmans 2021). Therefore, whether President Jokowi liked it or not, more restrictive public health policies were off the table.

With limited freedom of action, the Indonesian government relied on more gradual and selected lockdown measures, such as closing nonessential businesses and ordering workers to work from home. But even then the economic costs were substantial. According to the Indonesian MSME Association, more than thirty million of Indonesia's sixty-four million MSMEs were forced to close at various times, and around sixty million Indonesian workers did ultimately lose their jobs (Chew 2021). Once laid off, many workers returned from urban areas to their rural hometowns, which caused a further reduction in economic activity and a rise in poverty rates in cities. In addition, mobility and social gathering restrictions also affected supply chains and made raw materials more expensive. Indonesia already had higher import taxes, port service charges, and a variety of other fees and forms of red tape in comparison to neighboring countries. Thus, after lockdown measures against COVID-19 were implemented, MSMEs in the accommodation, food and beverage, tourism, transport, travel, and warehouse sectors were especially impacted (Atmojo and Fridayani 2021).

What kept the Indonesian economy afloat during the Asian financial crisis had thus become a structural defect in the COVID-19 pandemic. Due to these peculiar economic factors and costs, the Indonesian government could not adopt a more comprehensive and stringent policy program similar to the one in Malaysia. However, an important institutional factor also contributed to Indonesia's approach. Although the Indonesian government might be unitary in name, its decision-making structure on public health issues had already been decentralized over the archipelago (Hutchinson 2017; Lim et al. 2021). Indonesia grants regional and local governments varying degrees of decision-making autonomy in areas such as economic development, education, health, environment, and transportation (Pepinsky and Wihardja 2011; Nasution 2016; Talitha et al. 2020). In the public health sector specifically, significant resources and power had been transferred from the center to governments at lower levels over the past few decades (Mahendradhata et al. 2017; Miharti et al. 2016). The ambitious decentralization reform had produced mixed results, with pronounced structural problems of inequity (Rakmawati et al. 2019; Heywood and Choi 2010; Abdullah and Stoelwinder 2008). Indonesia's COVID-19 management reflected similar decentralizing patterns, with the central government delegating much of the responsibility to the provincial, municipal, and district governments (Meckelburg and Bal 2021; Sevindik et al. 2021; Fridayani and Soong 2021), leading to similarly inconsistent results (Adamy and Rani 2022). Therefore, Indonesia's institutional structure, while unitary, was permissive for the national executive to absent himself from stringent policymaking. Jokowi's Presidential Decree in March 2020 revealed his own intention to delegate decision-making power to lower levels of government in the first place, even long before a comprehensive national policy program against COVID-19 was being

6 PICK YOUR POISON: POLITICAL EXPEDIENCIES, ECONOMIC NECESSITIES... 139

debated. Without the central government's strong leadership, regional and local governments acted in the public health COVID-19 response by default, just as they did with other public health issues.

6.5 INDONESIA'S COVID-19 RESPONSE

Given the short-term political context and structural (economic) constraints, President Jokowi's reluctance to implement more stringent policy measures against COVID-19 and his refusal to declare a national state of emergency appears more rationalizable. The Indonesian government was in a stable political position, and Jokowi and his coalition enjoyed overwhelming popular support. There were no positive incentives for the government to implement drastic policies and disturb political normalcy. Jokowi and his government also preferred to preserve economic and social normalcy as much as possible, refusing to declare a national state of emergency, and only reluctantly agreed to a policy program that restricted business and social activities, albeit a mild and regionally focused one (Roziqin et al. 2021).

The first cases of COVID-19 in Indonesia were identified on March 2, 2020, when a 64-year-old woman and her 31-year-old daughter tested positive in West Java. By March 15, Indonesia had 117 confirmed cases, 5 of which were fatal. President Jokowi called on Indonesians to practice social distancing in order to slow the spread of COVID-19 (Olivia et al. 2020). While regional leaders in Jakarta, Banten, West Java, and other provinces had issued orders to close public areas, schools, and businesses, Jokowi had failed to declare a national state of emergency and announced that Indonesia would not pursue a full lockdown, criticizing regional leaders and health experts for suggesting it. Jokowi also came out in favor of so-called microrestrictions, which prevented local governments from imposing broader measures.

Jokowi's passive stance on the COVID-19 response soon became the center of a controversy. Health experts and independent observers called his policies reactive and contradictory to his image as an efficient leader when he was mayor of Solo and governor of Jakarta (Roziqin et al. 2021). They demanded that the central government impose national lockdowns, business closures, and restrictions on mass movement and social gatherings, especially when increasing evidence suggested that such measures could help contain the spread of COVID-19 (Fauzi and Paiman 2021). Senior ministers in his own cabinet, including Indonesia's top health official, encouraged Jokowi to take a more comprehensive and drastic approach. They advised that infection and death cases would spike dramatically if the government failed to implement stringent policy measures immediately. The adequate response, according to the ministers, would be to limit the movement of people, at least in the hardest hit areas.

On June 30, 2021, Jokowi met with business groups to discuss the possibility of a full-scale lockdown in Indonesia, but he encountered widespread resistance (Amul et al. 2022). Led by Indonesian Business Chamber of Commerce and Industry (Kadin) Chairman Rosan Roeslani, business groups pushed back against the recommendations of the senior ministers and health officials. They argued that stringent measures would stifle Indonesia's economic recovery and cause massive job losses. On the next day, Jokowi announced a formal policy program that included restrictions on mass movement and social gatherings but avoided full lockdowns (Olivia et al. 2020).

Soon after, Indonesia became the COVID-19 epicenter in Southeast Asia. According to data from the World Health Organization, daily infection rates in Indonesia doubled, and cases of fatality surpassed the rest of the world. Hospitals were overwhelmed, and only a small percentage of Indonesians were fully vaccinated. But even then, business interests refused to back down. New Kadin Chairman Arsjad Rasjid proposed a set of COVID-19 policy measures that allowed essential businesses to fully operate, nonessential businesses to operate at half-capacity, and economic aid for both businesses and workers. "Please don't take decisions that kill business or the economy because it will be very costly and dangerous for our social life," Rasjid told a group of reporters in Jakarta. "We understand that health is very important but we can't stop the economy totally" (Aditya and Heijmans 2021).

In his annual state-of-the-nation address in August 2021, Jokowi also reiterated his stance, stating that there was a need to strike a balance between health and economic interests amid the COVID-19 spike. "The pandemic has indeed significantly slowed down our economic growth, but it must not hinder the process of structural reforms of our economy," Jokowi told Parliament and the Indonesian public (Reuters 2021). He acknowledged the economic toll caused by the pandemic but said that "it must not hinder the process of structural reforms of our economy." The speech was given when Indonesia was seeing the highest number of cases of the highly lethal Delta variant. Like its counterpart in Malaysia, the Indonesian government had also faced strong criticism for its COVID-19 response policies, though for different reasons. "There is reluctance to take the bitter pill of restricting business," Achmad Sukarsono of global consulting firm Control Risks told Bloomberg News. "Indonesia is not using health specific considerations as the main reasoning behind their policies. It's more economic survival, and that comes from a lot of demand from people around the president, many of whom have businesses or are tied to businesses" (Aditya and Heijmans 2021).

Instead of implementing stringent policy measures such as lockdowns, therefore, Jokowi relied on vaccinations to contain the spread of the COVID-19 virus. He promised to distribute 181.5 million doses by the end of 2021. The general policy program adopted by the Indonesian government was called Large-Scale Social Restrictions (LSSR). It contained policy measures such as the closing of public areas and schools, limiting public transport, and restricting travel to and from certain regions. Unlike Malaysia's MCO, Indonesia's LSSR was mainly imposed by regional and local governments with the approval of the ministry of health at the central level. It was also less comprehensive and stringent (Olivia et al. 2020).

Even though the Jokowi government had transferred much decision-making power and resources to lower levels, letting provincial, municipal, and district governments decide when and how to implement response measures against the COVID-19 pandemic, it retained the power to block the more restrictive local measures. The Jokowi government frequently denied requests from lower-level governments to implement lockdowns. At the same time, Jokowi also tried to shift accountability and blame to lower-level governments. In June 2020, the presidential office published a rare video of a cabinet meeting in which Jokowi chastised his ministers for failing to take the COVID-19 pandemic seriously. He expressed direct anger toward the country's failure to adopt his Presidential Decree issued in March, which called on governors, regents, and mayors to act as chairpersons of the COVID-19 task force in their respective regions. According to Djayadi Hanan of Paramadina University, Jokowi was attempting to show the public that "We are trying very hard" so that "the public will not directly blame the president" (In-depth Creative, 2020). By "going public" with his anger and disappointment, Jokowi was shifting responsibility and blame to other Indonesian officials, in his own administration as well as at regional and local levels.

6.6 Conclusion

In this study, I have introduced a theoretical framework for understanding response policies to the COVID-19 pandemic and used it to assess the policy choices made by the governments in Malaysia and Indonesia. The focal point of this framework is the relationship between political expedience, economic necessities, and the level of policy stringency. With a slim majority in Parliament, an ongoing political crisis, and a prime minister who was often challenged for his undemocratic rise and frequent conflicts with coalition partners, the Malaysian government at the time had concrete political incentives to employ drastic strategies in order to suppress the opposition and stabilize itself. The pandemic provided Muhyiddin and his government the precise opportunity for doing so: a somewhat legitimate cause that could be used to keep opponents and voters at home. By declaring a national state of emergency and closing nonessential offices, the Muhyiddin government could temporarily suspend legislative and electoral processes, formulate and pass laws without oversight, and prevent opponents from mobilizing and challenging its rule. In other words, the Muhyiddin government's fight against COVID-19 was also a story about its political survival. Nevertheless, the implementation of these measures also required a robust economy to absorb the cost of lockdowns, closures, and other restrictions. While not as advanced as Western countries, Malaysia's economy was still relatively well structured and its workforce well supported. These comparative advantages expanded the range of policy choices and ultimately enabled the Muhyiddin government to implement a set of stringent policies—in particular the national state of emergency—that served its own political interests.

Indonesia's COVID-19 policy response, on the other hand, was quite different. The president and his government enjoyed overwhelming majority support and were in strong political positions. There was no need to employ drastic strategies and change the status quo. President Jokowi's preference was to govern the country as it was. But even if the Jokowi government desired stringent policy measures, Indonesia's economy limited its set of policy options. More specifically, the Indonesian economy was not structured well and its workforce not supported well enough to absorb the exceedingly high costs of stringent policy measures. It was dominated by MSMEs that could not easily adjust to drastic social and economic changes. Millions of jobs had been lost and potential revenues evaporated. As a result, the Jokowi government avoided implementing stringent policy measures as much as possible. The public health consequences were severe, as many Indonesians might have been infected with the COVID-19 virus as a result of the lackluster effort at containing the virus. Nonetheless, the Jokowi government worried that if stringent policy measures were widely and thoroughly implemented, the economic and social costs for Indonesians could be even higher. For these reasons, Indonesia chose a more conservative and regional-based response option.

REFERENCES

Abdullah, A. and Stoelwinder, J. (2008) Decentralization and health resource allocation: a case study at the district level in Indonesia. *Healthcare Quarterly* (Toronto, Ont.), 11(2), pp. 117–125.

Adamy, A. and Rani, H. A. (2022) An evaluation of community satisfaction with the government's COVID-19 pandemic response in Aceh, Indonesia. *International Journal of Disaster Risk Reduction*, 69, 102723.

Aditya, A. and Heijmans, P. (2021) 'How anti-lockdown elites swayed Jokowi, fueling Indonesia crisis', *Bloomberg News*, 21 July.

Amul, G. G., Ang, M., Kraybill, D., Ong, S. E. and Yoong, J. (2022) 'Responses to COVID-19 in southeast Asia: diverse paths and ongoing challenges', *Asian Economic Policy Review*, 17(1), pp. 90–110.

Arnakim, L. Y. and Kibtiah, T. M. (2021) 'Response of ASEAN member states to the spread of COVID-19 in southeast Asia', *IOP Conference Series: Earth and Environmental Science*.

Atmojo, M. E. and Fridayani, H. D. (2021) 'An assessment of Covid-19 pandemic impact on Indonesian tourism sector', *Journal of Governance and Public Policy*, 8(1).

Dingel, J. I. and Neiman, B. (2020) 'How many jobs can be done at home?', *Journal of Public Economics*, 189.

Chew, Amy. (2021) 'Covid-19 cost 60 million Indonesians their jobs in MSMEs. Can its economic "hero" recover?' *South China Morning Post*, 3 September.

Djalante, R., Lassa, J., Setiamarga, D., Sudjatma, A., Indrawan, M., Haryanto, B., ... and Warsilah, H. (2020) Review and analysis of current responses to COVID-19 in Indonesia: Period of January to March 2020. *Progress in Disaster Science*, 6, 100091.

Fauzi, M. A. and Paiman, N. (2021) 'COVID-19 pandemic in southeast Asia: intervention and mitigation efforts', *Asian Education and Development Studies*, 10(2), pp. 176–184.

Fridayani, H. D. and Soong, J. J. (2021) The emergent role of local government on COVID-19 outbreak in Indonesia: A new state-society perspective. *Journal of Governance*, 6(1), pp. 23–45.

Hashim, J. H., Adman, M. A., Hashim, Z., Radi, M. F. M. and Kwan, S. C. (2021) 'COVID-19 epidemic in Malaysia: epidemic progression, challenges, and response', *Frontiers in Public Health*, 9.

Heywood, P. and Choi, Y. (2010) Health system performance at the district level in Indonesia after decentralization. *BMC International Health and Human Rights*, 10(1), pp. 1–12.

Hutchinson, F. E. (2017) '(De)centralization and the missing middle in Indonesia and Malaysia', *Sojourn: Journal of Social Issues in Southeast Asia*, 32(2), pp. 291–335.

In-depth Creative. (2020) 'E47: Local, Central & the Blame Game with Dr. Djayadi Hanan.'

Khatiwada, S., El Achkar Hilal, S., Arao, R. M. and Generalao, I. N. (2021) 'COVID-19 and labor markets in southeast Asia: evidence from Indonesia, Malaysia, the Philippines, Thailand, and Viet Nam', *Asian Development Bank*.

Lim, G., Li, C. and Syailendra, E. A. (2021) 'Why is it so hard to push Chinese railway projects in Southeast Asia? The role of domestic politics in Malaysia and Indonesia', *World Development*, 138.

Ling, G. H. T., et al. (2021) 'Factors influencing Asia-Pacific countries' success level in curbing COVID-19: a review using a social-ecological system (SES) framework', *International Journal of Environmental Research and Public Health*, 18(4), pp. 1704.

Mahendradhata, Y., et al. (2017) 'The republic of Indonesia health system review', *Health Systems in Transition*, 7(1).

Meckelburg, R. and Bal, C. S. (2021) Indonesia and Covid-19: Decentralization and social conflict. In *Covid-19 and governance* (pp. 74–87). Routledge.

Miharti, S., Holzhacker, R. L. and Wittek, R. (2016) Decentralization and primary health care innovations in Indonesia. *Decentralization and Governance in Indonesia*, pp. 53–78.

Department of Statistics Malaysia. (2020) *Report of Special Survey on Effects of COVID-19 on Economy & Individual—Round 1.*

Nasution, A. (2016) 'The government decentralization program in Indonesia', *Asian Development Bank Institute Working Paper Series.*

Olivia, S., Gibson, J. and Nasrudin, R. (2020) 'Indonesia in the time of Covid-19', *Bulletin of Indonesian Economic Studies*, 56(2), pp. 143–174.

Pepinsky, T. B. and Wihardja, M. M. (2011) 'Decentralization and economic performance in Indonesia', *Journal of East Asian Studies*, 11(3), pp. 337–371.

Rahman, A. A., Jasmin, A. F. and Schmillen, A. (2020) 'The vulnerability of jobs to COVID-19: the case of Malaysia', *Yusof Ishak Institute Working Paper.*

Rakmawati, T., Hinchcliff, R. and Pardosi, J. F. (2019) 'District-level impacts of health system decentralization in Indonesia: a systematic review', *The*

International Journal of Health Planning and Management, 34(2), pp. 1026–1053.

Ratcliffe, R. (2021) 'Malaysia declares Covid state of emergency amid political turmoil', *The Guardian*, 12 January.

Reuters. (2021) 'Indonesia president says need to balance health and economy in pandemic', *Reuters*, 16 August.

Roziqin, A., Mas'udi, S. Y. F. and Sihidi, I. T. (2021) 'An analysis of Indonesian government policies against COVID-19', *Public Administration and Policy: An Asia-Pacific Journal*, 24(1), pp. 92–107.

Sevindik, I., Tosun, M. S. and Yilmaz, S. (2021) Local response to the covid-19 pandemic: The case of Indonesia. *Sustainability*, 13(10), 5620.

Talitha, T., Firman, T. and Hudalah, D. (2020) 'Welcoming two decades of decentralization in Indonesia: a regional development perspective', *Territory, Politics, Governance*, 8(5), pp. 690–708.

Toshkov, D., Carroll, B. and Yesilkagit, K. (2021) 'Government capacity, societal trust or party preferences: what accounts for the variety of national policy responses to the COVID-19 pandemic in Europe?', *Journal of European Public Policy*, 29(7), pp. 1009–1028.

CHAPTER 7

Populist Responses to COVID-19: Turkey and Israel as Cases of Proscience Populism and the United States and Brazil as Examples of Science-Skeptic Populism

Mert Can Bayar and Didem Seyis

7.1 Introduction

The COVID-19 pandemic came as a significant and politically dangerous surprise for governments worldwide. Where countries were readying for the elections or battling economic or constitutional crises, the COVID-19 pandemic caught political and social systems unguarded and most vulnerable. As of 2022, nearly two and a half years after patient zero was announced, the total of COVID-19 cases worldwide is nearing 550 million, with more than 6 million reported deaths, while the World Health Organization's (WHO) excess mortality data estimates have reached almost 15 million deaths worldwide for 2020 and 2021 combined (World

---

M. C. Bayar (✉) • D. Seyis
Department of Political Science, Binghamton University,
Binghamton, NY, USA
e-mail: mbayar1@binghamton.edu; dseyis1@binghamton.edu

© The Author(s), under exclusive license to Springer Nature
Switzerland AG 2023
O. Shvetsova (ed.), *Government Responses to the COVID-19 Pandemic*, https://doi.org/10.1007/978-3-031-30844-4_7

147

Health Organization 2022). Most governments responded to this global health crisis by collaborating with expert-led teams and learning from each other's practices, looking for the best ways to diminish its impacts (Shvetsova et al. 2020). To contain the pandemic, they had to implement harsh protective policies such as border closures, mandatory quarantines, lockdowns, mask mandates, closure of public areas, and restrictions on individual mobility (Shvetsova et al. 2022). In short, governments were under immense pressure to implement unpopular, economically costly, and expert-advised policy decisions.

Not surprisingly, populist governments do not top the list when we consider the implementation of unpopular and expert-advised decisions. These are difficult and costly policies, and populist leaders/parties claim to be the voice of the general will and are strongly anti-expert (Kavakli 2020; Seyis 2021; Bayerlein et al. 2021; Naushirvanov et al. 2022). Thus, many pundits and scholars believed the pandemic would be the end of populism as we know it (Mounk 2021; Laudicina 2021; Foa et al. 2022). In support of this expectation, we saw the Trump administration unseated in the USA, Netanyahu lose his seat after a decade in Israel, Bolsonaro polling fifteen points lower than his closest rival (Luiz Inácio "Lula" da Silva) on the eve of Brazil's presidential elections, and Erdogan polling his lowest since he came to power in Turkey in 2002. Yet we argue that a sort of populism that we rarely consider did survive the pandemic.

Contrary to expectations, not all populists took an anti-expert, science-skeptic discourse toward the pandemic. For instance, Erdogan of Turkey, one of the most prominent populists of our time, took the pandemic seriously, avoiding misinformation and conspiracy theories surrounding the pandemic (masks and social distancing in particular and protective policies in general) (Seyis 2021). Instead, he put forth a proscience discourse overall and delegated most of his immense presidential power in handling the pandemic to the experts, namely, to his minister of health and a medical doctor, Dr. Fahrettin Koca.[1]

Another proscience populist was Netanyahu of Israel. Netanyahu's government also took the pandemic seriously, implementing one of the harshest nation-wide protective policy packages throughout 2020

---

[1] It is important to note that we acknowledge the fact that there surely are political calculations behind Erdogan's delegation of power to the minister of health. By delegating power, he also delegated possible blames for failure. He played it safe and tried to protect his positive image among his constituency by not being in the spotlight during the crisis.

(Shvetsova et al. 2022; Maor et al. 2020). He assembled a small team within his government and led the crisis response to the pandemic, informing citizens himself through television and took the opportunity to frame the crisis in ways that benefited his government's survival.

On the other hand, such populist presidents as Donald Trump and Jair Bolsonaro have downplayed the importance of the COVID-19 pandemic: making parallels with the flu (Phillips 2020a; Bump 2020), claiming that it will pass in a few months (Wolfe and Dale 2020), refusing to wear masks in public (Cathey 2020; Pazzanese 2020), refusing to implement mask mandates (Firozi 2020; Victor et al. 2020) and social distancing protocols (Perez 2020; Ramsay 2021; Human Rights Watch 2020), organizing mass rallies nationwide (Brito and Fonseca 2021; Ray 2022), sabotaging provincial/state-level implementation of protective measures (VanDusky-Allen et al. 2020; Cheatham 2020), and mocking government officials who implemented such policies (Cathey 2020; Phillips 2020b). We call this type of populist response science-skeptic populism.

In this chapter, we demonstrate a powerful yet undervalued variation in populist governance revealed during the COVID-19 pandemic: proscience vs. science-skeptic populism. Using our Protective Policy Index (PPI) dataset (Shvetsova et al. 2022), composed of the most salient protective policies and behaviors used by populist governments such as lockdowns, mask mandates, and social distancing requirements (for a detailed description see Chap. 1), we show how Israel and Turkey under Netanyahu and Erdogan, respectively, represent a proscience populism within which these leaders took the pandemic seriously and responded to the pandemic with a proexpert and proscience discourse.[2] We contrast this with policy and behavior among other populists such as Donald Trump and Jair Bolsonaro who responded with science-skeptic populism and are inherently anti-expert. The types of populism identified here are not limited to these four countries and their leaders. These cases are merely illustrative examples of right-wing populist leadership that goes beyond our case studies. We argue that this distinction is a fundamental difference between these two types of populism, and it stems from the demand side of populism: constituent expectations. Whereas Bolsonaro and Trump built their winning coalitions on a radical right-wing mobilization with science-skeptic and anti-expert constituencies, Erdogan and Netanyahu built their winning

---

[2] For exceptions to this generalization of proscience attitudes of Erdogan and Netanyahu, please see our last paragraph in the alternative explanations section.

coalitions with their partners in the center (right and left) that are neither science-skeptic nor anti-expert per se.

Israel and Turkey are our cases of proscience populism, and we discuss the contextual factors that restricted or magnified their governments' responses to the pandemic. Before the pandemic, these two countries were both engulfed in a major crisis that surprisingly differentiated their responses to the pandemic. Erdogan's Turkey was battling an immense economic crisis following a recession, and Netanyahu's caretaker government was undergoing a political and constitutional crisis, Netanyahu's corruption trial, and a series of indecisive elections. In short, Erdogan's economic vulnerability led his government to underreact to the pandemic, even though he took the crisis seriously at the discursive level (Seyis 2021; Laebens and Ozturk 2022). On the other hand, Netanyahu's political and constitutional crisis led his government to disproportionately overreact to the pandemic in terms of the extent to which they implemented protective policies (Maor et al. 2020).

The remainder of this chapter is organized as follows. We first explain our conceptualization of populism and discuss how the COVID-19 pandemic unveiled a science-related variation in populist government behavior. Then we introduce our case studies in detail and present the findings from our original extensive PPI dataset. In conclusion, we present alternative explanations and the limitations of this analysis.

7.2   Populist Responses to the Pandemic: Proscience Populism and Science-Skeptic Populism

Although the COVID-19 pandemic caught all governments off guard, some followed scientific opinion closer than others and swiftly introduced public health restrictions in compliance with the instructions of global health authorities such as the WHO. Countries such as South Korea, Japan, Canada, and Australia are among those who took the pandemic seriously and introduced stringent policies (and diligently enforced them) to contain and control the spread of COVID-19 in line with the advice of scientists. These countries quickly introduced stringent protective policies such as border closures, school and entertainment venue closures, and quarantine requirements after travel and testing requirements and kept them in place for a long time (Adeel et al. 2020; Shvetsova et al. 2020, 2022). While these nonpopulist governments have closely followed scientific advice in combatting the pandemic, populist governments in the USA, Brazil, Mexico, and Nicaragua downplayed the pandemic and objected to health experts' warnings and suggestions. But are all populists so prone to rejecting expert opinion?

In this chapter, we use Cas Mudde's definition of populism as a thin-centered ideology that separates society into two homogeneous yet antagonistic groups, "the pure people" and "the corrupt elite," and that sees politics as an expression of the general will of the people (Mudde 2004). Put simply, populism is an ideology that glorifies the so-called general will (of the "pure people") and dislikes any checks and limitations on the "will of the people." Therefore, populists are inherently antiestablishment, anti-elitist, and, for that matter, anti-expert, as well as science-sceptic. Hence, the populist ideology provides a solid basis for populist governments to reject expert opinion to combat the pandemic on the grounds that it is not "the will of the people" (Huber 2020; Staerklé et al. 2022). As a result, it is not very shocking to see many scholars argue that populist governments' healthcare policy responses have been, on average, different from those of mainstream governments irrespective of whether populists are right-wing or left-wing[3] (Meyer 2020; Seyis 2021; Bayerlein et al. 2021; Naushirvanov et al. 2022).

Even though scholars classify leaders and governments as populist or nonpopulist or antipopulist (Mudde 2017), government behavior during the COVID-19 crisis was shaped by such constraining contextual pressures as economic recession, loss of public support for the government, weakening governing coalitions, constituents' existing attitudes toward experts and science, and their perception of the COVID-19 threat (Shvetsova et al. 2020, 2021, 2022; Brubaker 2021). Furthermore, the opportunity structures, such as the political mechanisms of unitary and centralized systems of government, as opposed to federal governance or health care, influenced populists' choices of public health policy strategy (Shvetsova et al. 2020; VanDusky-Allen et al. 2020; Adeel et al. 2020;

---

[3] Populists are anti-elitist and anti-expert irrespective of their ideological position on the political spectrum. Examples of populist governments also lend support to the approach that ideology did not prove a strong predictor of populist governments' pandemic response. We should also note that most populist incumbents during the height of the pandemic were right-wing. Among the few left-wing populist incumbents, some took the pandemic seriously (e.g., Nicolás Maduro in Venezuela and Rodrigo Duterte in Philippines), while others downplayed it (Andrés Manuel López Obrador in Mexico and Daniel Ortega in Nicaragua) (Meyer 2020).

Shvetsova et al. 2021). In this chapter, we limit our focus to constituency expectations (demand) and important contextual factors (constraints) that we suggest drove the variation in populist leaders' strategies.

7.2.1 What Their Constituency Expects Determines Populists' Responses

Trump, Bolsonaro, Erdogan, and Netanyahu all have relatively radical-right core constituencies, yet the radicalism in their constituencies differs greatly. For Trump's core constituency, the American radical right, the most salient issues include immigration, science, and expert denial such as climate change denial (Dietz 2020), evolution denial (Miller et al. 2022), and the infamous vaccination-autism controversy (Miller 2015; Buncombe 2018). White Evangelical voters, who have the highest antivaccine attitudes according to Pew Research, are among Trump's core constituency (Concoran et al. 2021). Similarly, Bolsonaro's core constituency has both radical-right and illiberal values (Castanho Silva et al. 2022). Like Trump, Bolsonaro has strong support from science-skeptic Evangelical Protestant voters, the majority of whom also deny evolution and climate change (Veldman 2019; Deutsche Welle 2020). However, Erdogan's core constituency is the most pro-immigration/refugee in the Turkish population (Erdogan and Semerci 2018) and not statistically different from the rest of the electorate in their attitudes toward science (Erisen 2022). Further, a recent study showed that climate change skepticism as well as COVID-19 skepticism was correlated more with the left than the right in Turkey (Enders et al. 2022).

Skepticism about COVID-19 is more visible in the right wing of the USA and Brazil. A study on science skepticism conducted in twenty-four countries found that political conservatism in Israel and Turkey did not predict climate change skepticism, whereas it did in the USA and Brazil (Rutjens et al. 2022). Similarly, the vaccine hesitancy in Israel and Turkey does not depend on science literacy, whereas it does in the United States and Brazil. This means that there is a broad societal consensus on vaccine safety in Israel and Turkey, whereas this consensus in the USA and Brazil is fragile and depends on individual factors such as science literacy. In the USA, Republicans are almost twice as likely as Democrats to say that COVID-19 is not a major health threat to Americans (Deane et al. 2021) and four times more likely to say that the COVID-19 crisis is exaggerated (Mitchell et al. 2021). Only 29% of Republicans vis-a-vis 64% of Democrats

7 POPULIST RESPONSES TO COVID-19: TURKEY AND ISRAEL AS CASES... 153

said that people should always wear a mask, only 49% of Republicans compared to 69% of Democrats said that social distancing reduced the spread of the disease (Funk and Tyson 2020).[4]

This skepticism on the American and Brazilian right is not limited to COVID-19. According to a Pew survey from 2019, only 34% of Republicans agreed that scientific experts made better science-related policy decisions than other people (Funk 2020). Only 37% of conservative Republicans that are part of former President Trump's core constituency believe that scientists understand the causes of climate change. Among the same group, only 36% think that scientists know the right way to address climate change and, most strikingly, only 14% of conservative Republicans say human activity contributes a great deal to climate change (Funk and Hefferon 2019). In short, Erdogan's and Netanyahu's constituencies expected quite the opposite of what Trump's and Bolsonaro's expected for their leaders to deliver. During the pandemic, for Trump and Bolsonaro supporters, the most important issue has been their freedom to choose, but for Erdogan and Netanyahu supporters, the most important issue is safety and security.[5]

It is crucial to note here that there are important exceptions to this proscience attitude of Erdogan and Netanyahu. The first one concerns evolutionary theory. Turkish and Israeli biology curriculums largely avoid teaching evolution as a legitimate scientific theory that has surpassed centuries-old falsification trials. They ignore the theory as a whole and tell educators to focus on other topics (Duran 2017; Staff 2018; BBC News Turkish 2021; France24 2020).[6] One study found that religious

---

[4] It is crucial to note that the partisan divide was there before the pandemic in terms of science skepticism and trust in experts, yet the COVID-19 pandemic widened the gap on many fronts due to the science-skeptic politics endorsed by former President Trump and the GOP. It should also be noted that the most radical and science-denialist portion of American society, Evangelicals, became increasingly important within the Republican Party over the years, and that also has had a major impact on the radical turn of the Republican Party. In the 1970s, Republicans were more confident about science than religion (O'Brien and Noy 2020).

[5] We should note that this can also be understood as a framing choice by the elite. Trump and Bolsonaro played the pandemic as a discussion of freedom versus tyranny of restrictions that are the protective policies, whereas Netanyahu and Erdogan framed it as a national security issue, where they need every one of their citizens to obey the rules like they have been required to do by their security-oriented states for decades.

[6] Another counterexample to our generalization of Erdogan's and Netanyahu's proscience attitude and discourse is the fact that both leaders organized rallies and endorsed public gatherings in closed quarters (for political and/or religious purposes) during the pandemic.

orthodoxy in Turkey and Israel (as well as US and Brazil) was a strong predictor of evolution skepticism that could be considered a proxy indicator of science skepticism beyond COVID-19 (Rutjens et al. 2022). The second exception concerns Erdogan's attitude toward the Turkish Medical Association (TMA) during the first year of the pandemic (Cupolo 2020a). Erdogan constantly threatened the association and accused it of terrorism due to the association's public hearings about the underreported case and death numbers (Cupolo 2020b). Later, the ministry of health admitted the underreporting of COVID case numbers (Cupolo 2020c), vindicating the TMA. In short, even though Erdogan and Netanyahu put forth a pro-science attitude during the crisis, their approaches carry notable caveats of science skepticism in general and in the COVID-19 pandemic in particular.

7.2.2 Erdogan and Netanyahu: Reformed Radicals Making Their Careers in the Center

Even though both Netanyahu and Erdogan began their political careers as antiestablishment and radical-right figures within antiestablishment and radical-right parties, their luck in government came when they turned toward the center and became less antiestablishment and more compromise-oriented (Mitchell 2015; Cagaptay 2020). During Erdogan's first election campaign before the 2002 elections in which he came to power, Erdogan infamously stated that he moved away from the party's Islamist roots and grew into a moderate center-right politician (Bolukbasi 2012). This move toward the center, at least on the discursive level, lasted until mid-2010s (Laebens and Ozturk 2021) and held together the center-right support for Erdogan's single-party government for more than a decade within Turkey's traditionally factionalized political environment with a proportional electoral system and 10 percent electoral threshold.

Netanyahu, on the other hand, came to government various times over the course of twenty-five years and formed coalitions with both centrist and center-left parties. As a radical yet flexible figure, he did not hesitate to compromise and collaborate with the other side of the aisle (Peleg 2019). This flexibility and turn toward the center enabled both politicians to form grand coalitions. This flexibility required reliance on the center vote, unlike other populists such as Donald Trump and Jair Bolsonaro. Both Trump and Bolsonaro became incumbents as radical right-wing populists who built their entire platform on an antiestablishment, conspiracist, and populist radical-right politics (Neiwert 2017; Renno 2020). Thus, even though the core constituency of these four leaders can be considered radical on the generic ideological spectrum, the momentum that made their careers came in different contexts with different coalitions. For Erdogan and Netanyahu, it was the coalition with the center that made them come to and stay in power, but for Trump and Bolsonaro, it was the mobilization of the radical right-wing, antiestablishment voters that propelled them to power.

7.3   PROTECTIVE POLICY INDEX MEASURE AND FINDINGS

Proscience and science-skeptic populists varied in the ways in which they responded to the pandemic. The most important factors that reveal this variation are the opposite approaches these two types of populists took when it came to mask mandates, lockdowns, and other protective measures. Thus, our PPI dataset is a valuable asset to examine the populist governments' responses to the COVID-19 pandemic, explore the proscience populist approach, and further analyze the similarities and differences between the two types of populist government response identified in this chapter.

Figure 7.1 shows the national/federal-level PPI computed based only on the policies of national governments (thus excluding the policy contributions of regional governments)[7] throughout 2020 in Brazil, Israel, Turkey, and the United States. Public health protective policies originated in each country around mid-March 2020, with the COVID-19 cases increasing worldwide during the first wave. During the summer of 2020, the national measures eased in Israel and Turkey and remained constant in Brazil and the United States. Of the four countries, the national governments in Israel and Turkey responded to the pandemic with the most stringent measures. Although all four leaders and their governments are considered populists, these results support our hypothesis that there is meaningful variation in populists' responses to the COVID-19 pandemic at both the discursive and ground level.

---

[7] For more information on the COVID-19 PPI dataset, please see Shvetsova et al. (2022).

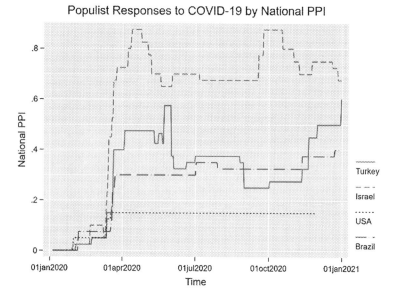

Fig. 7.1 Daily national (federal) PPI in Brazil, Israel, Turkey, and USA, year 2020. (Here we use national/federal PPI rather than total since our argument relies on national/federal level of responses to the pandemic. For a comparison and discussion on the national versus total PPI, please refer to the online appendix.) (Source: Shvetsova et al. 2022)

7.4 THE CASE OF ISRAEL: DISPROPORTIONATE MEASURES IN A "NATIONAL SECURITY" CRISIS

Among the four, Israel leads in applying the most stringent protective policies against the COVID-19 pandemic, with a mean 2020 national PPI of 0.70 starting from March 1, 2020. That the Israeli government possibly even overreacted, due to political motives, was evident during Rosh Hashana, the Jewish New Year, when synagogues are traditionally overcrowded (starting from September 18) (Maor et al. 2020). Israel's rather high national PPI mean of 0.70 and the pattern of policy implementation demonstrate how the Netanyahu government perceived and framed the pandemic as a national security issue rather than a health crisis and used the crisis for political means—to pursue the survival of their caretaker

Table 7.1 Comparison of Regime Type, Government Strength, and GDP per capita in Brazil, Israel, Turkey, and USA

Country	Regime Type	Δ in Gov't Strength 2019–2016	Δ in Gov't Strength 2020–2019	Δ in GDP Per Capita 2019–2016	Δ in GDP Per Capita 2020–2019
Israel	Unitary/ Par	-3.42%	0.63%	6847	226
Turkey	Unitary/ Pres.	-6.95%	-8%	-908	-585
Brazil	Federal/ Pres.	NA	-0.39%	-1914	-2101
USA	Federal/ Pres.	NA	NA	5185	-2073

Sources: World Bank (2022), "GDP Per Capita (US$)". "Δ in Gov't Strength" stands for change in government strength. The percentages in government strength are calculated by the change in vote shares of the government party or coalitions. Under the regime type column, "Par." stands for parliamentary system and "Pres." for presidential system. NA stands for not available (since Brazil's Bolsonaro government did not come to power till 2018. We noted its February 19, 2016, performance as missing (NA). We chose to keep the USA missing as well because it is difficult to identify government strength with party vote in the USA.)

government. Due to its relative economic stability before and during the pandemic (as shown in Table 7.1), Israel was capable of implementing unpopular and stringent nationwide policies. The Netanyahu government used the favorable pretext of security and economic stability to disproportionately react to the COVID-19 pandemic and further the survival of the government as well as delay Netanyahu's corruption trial.

As the Netanyahu government suffered from a parliamentary gridlock within a constitutional crisis and a corruption trial for the prime minister, Netanyahu's party suffered a 3.42% loss from the 2015 to the 2019 elections. Their coalition's vote share declined from 48% to 45%. In the Israeli at-large proportional parliamentary system, this was a game-changing loss that enabled a possible opposition majority in the Knesset. Furthermore, the parliamentary opposition was more unified than ever and ready to strike against Netanyahu's government on multiple battlefields (constitutional, judicial, and political) (BBC News 2021).

Netanyahu pursued the survival of his weakening coalition and managed the crisis by prioritizing political considerations (Boin et al. 2020). Maor et al. (2020) described Israel's response to the pandemic as a "deliberate disproportionate policy response." They argued that in the first months of the pandemic, Netanyahu employed a policy of overreaction at the rhetorical level in his daily televised speeches to the public (Gesser-Edelsburg and Hijazi 2020), seizing the "creeping crisis" (Boin et al. 2020) by making parallels between the plagues of medieval Europe and the COVID-19 pandemic and even using the Holocaust as an example to describe the severity of the crisis (Gesser-Edelsburg and Hijazi 2020). Gesser-Edelsburg and Hijazi (2020) argued that this was a deliberate move by Netanyahu to create a sense of fear and unify the country under his centralized leadership. In line with this argument, Netanyahu offered an "emergency unity government" to the main opposition party leader, Benny Gantz, in a move that extended his prime ministership for a year.[8]

On the other hand, the Israeli economy was doing relatively well compared with the other countries that we investigate here. This economic stability and prosperity provided the Israeli government with the capability to implement economically costly protective measures. As shown in Table 7.2, the country's GDP per capita had been rising before the pandemic. Despite slowing during the pandemic, the GDP growth did not drop below zero, unlike in many advanced economies (Pardhan and Drydakis 2021).[9]

---

[8] Despite Netanyahu's tough rhetoric, on the ground, his response was tailored to his constituency's needs (Waitzberg et al. 2020). Since thousands of Israeli students and Ultra-Orthodox Jewish families were returning to Israel from New York, his government could not close the border with the USA at a time in which the USA, and specifically New York City, was the epicenter of the pandemic. Further, during the Passover holiday, the same constituency considerations led Netanyahu and his team to a deliberate policy overreaction, enforcing a national curfew even though the epidemiological data pointed out that a differential response covering in particular Ultra-Orthodox localities, which were hotspots for the spread of the virus, should have been implemented (Maor et al. 2020). This tailored policy response had two purposes: to ease off the constituency pressure by prioritizing their needs over those of the country as a whole.

[9] Level of democracy is an important factor that we did not include in Tables 7.1 or 7.2. The literature suggests that, contrary to expectations, democracies did a better job at protecting their citizens than did nondemocracies (Shvetsova et al. 2020). Yet Freedom House ratings and Polity IV scores show that Israel (Freedom House: 76/100, Polity IV (2018): 6/10), the United States (83/100, 8/10), and Brazil (73/100, 8/10) are considered free and democratic, whereas Turkey (32/100, -4/10) is considered not free, which does not reflect its level of response. Therefore, we consider the national response to COVID-19 as not stemming from the level of political rights, civil liberties, or overall level of democracy in these four cases.

7.5 The Case of Turkey: Economic Vulnerability and Underreaction in Protective Policies

Turkey's National PPI in 2020 averaged 0.36, barely above that of Brazil's (see Table 7.2 for details). Erdogan's government was unable to implement necessary policies in full form since such policies threatened serious short-term economic impact for the most vulnerable households, Erdogan's core electoral supporters (Selcuki 2021). Rather than implementing preemptive lockdowns during the peak of the first wave, the government chose to implement weekend curfews and stay-at-home orders for the over-65 and under-18 populations (Seyis 2021). As seen in Fig. 7.1, Turkey further eased the protective policies during the summer of 2020 because of the dependence of the Turkish economy on international tourism. The sudden decrease in national PPI in September 2020 reflected the government's decision to open schools in the fall, enabling parents to keep their jobs. Starting from November 2020, Turkey gradually increased the protective measures again, and at the end of the year, the national PPI approached 0.6, rising to the level of Israel's.

The Turkish economy has been in serious trouble since the regime change and the introduction of the presidential system in 2017. The COVID-19 pandemic struck the Turkish economy when it was in a vulnerable state and suffering from a recession. Turkish GDP per capita started to decline after its 2013 peak ($12,614 in 2013) and has been in

Table 7.2 Comparison of National and Total PPI, Mortality, and Healthcare Institutions in Brazil, Israel, Turkey, and USA

Country	National PPI	Total PPI	Reported Mortality/Pp 2020	Excess Mortality/Pp 2020	Universal Healthcare	Primarily Resp. for Healthcare
Israel	0.70 (0.15)	0.70 (0.15)	36.2	28 (7)	Yes	Central Gov't
Turkey	0.36 (0.11)	0.37 (0.12)	24.5	150 (21)	Yes	Central Gov't
Brazil	0.31 (0.07)	0.56 (0.12)	90.6	99 (4)	Yes	Regional Gov't
USA	0.15 (0.02)	0.52 (0.12)	106.9	141 (9)	No	Central Gov't

Sources: Shvetsova et al. (2022). World Health Organization, "COVID Excess Deaths". "Pp" stands for per 100.000 population.

freefall since that time. During the pandemic, the Turkish economy continued sinking and lost an additional $565 per capita to the rising inflation and devaluation of the Turkish lira. Even though Erdogan took the pandemic seriously, he was politically constrained from implementing the most economically costly and unpopular public health measures. For instance, though a ban on Friday prayers was introduced on March 16, 2020, Erdogan's regime hesitated to continue the closure of mosques and reinstated communal Friday prayers on May 29, 2020, with social distancing mandates in place (BBC News Turkish 2020). His government simply did not have the political capital to implement the more stringent protective measures, such as preemptive lockdowns and closures of superspreader areas like mosques and shopping malls.

As the WHO's excess mortality data show (Table 7.2), government's trade-off on protective measures, calculating the political costs for government survival, led Turkey to pay a steep price in mortality (BBC News Turkish 2022). Notice that out of the four countries exmined in this chapter, Turkey's mortality reporting was by far the least transparent: based on the difference between reported mortality and WHO's excess mortality projections, Turkey reported only one out of five COVID-19-related deaths in 2020 (World Health Organization 2022; Kisa and Kisa 2020.

Even though Erdogan was not in an immediate political crisis like Netanyahu, he was suffering from the same disease: a weakening coalition. His governing party lost 7 percent of its national support in three years (2016 to 2019) and lost 8 percent during the pandemic (from 38 to 30 percent), the lowest it has been since Erdogan came to power in 2002 (34 percent). Unlike Netanyahu, Erdogan did not have the economic cushion or the popular salience of the security issue to enforce unpopular and costly protective policies to reconsolidate his power. Thus, his strategy focused on blame avoidance and suppression of real COVID-19 cases and mortality statistics. He delegated announcements of the daily COVID-19 numbers to his minister of health, Dr. Fahrettin Koca, whereas Netanyahu made such announcements personally. Erdogan aimed to avoid taking the blame for probable failures, whereas Netanyahu wanted the glory of a possible success in handling the public health crisis. Thus, battling an economic crisis led to Turkey's relative underreaction in pursuing protective measures. This underreaction cost Turkey the highest excess mortality rate in 2020 among the four countries analyzed here (see Table 7.2 for details).

7.6 Brazil and the United States as Examples of Science-Skeptic Populism

Brazil and the USA offer illustrations of how science-skeptic populist leadership can willfully underreact, on both the discursive and policy levels, to an existential crisis. President Donald Trump's outspoken skepticism over the effectiveness of masks despite the firm stance of Dr. Anthony Fauci, the Director of the National Institute of Allergy and Infectious Diseases (NIAID) and the Centers for Disease Control and Prevention (CDC) (Zimmer 2020). The former president even mocked his opponent Joe Biden during the presidential debate for always wearing a mask during his campaign (CNN 2020a). As expected from these examples, the United States did not introduce highly stringent policy measures at the national/ federal level (Adeel et al. 2020).

The former US president's indifference, if not opposition, to mask wearing was not without a reason. This stance against COVID-19 protective measures was reflective of his supporters' attitudes. According to exit polls during the 2020 US elections, only 35% of Trump supporters saw mask wearing in public as a public health responsibility, whereas this figure was 64% among Biden voters (CNN 2020b). Widespread protests across the USA by Trump supporters against mask mandates and stay-at-home orders confirmed the resistance to the pandemic restrictions in the poll findings (Stewart 2020; Andone 2020). Trump supporters' strong opposition to COVID-19 restrictions along with the former president's populist drive to reflect "the will of the people" explain why Trump's government refrained from introducing stringent protective policies on the national level and placed most of the burden of the pandemic response to subnational governments (Adeel et al. 2020; Shvetsova et al. 2021).

The pandemic response of the Brazilian government under Jair Bolsonaro was similar to that of the Trump administration. Despite warnings from scientists and experts, President Bolsonaro commented that COVID-19 was no more than "a little flu" and that the seriousness of the pandemic was being exaggerated by the opposition and the media to plot against the Bolsonaro administration (Phillips 2020a). Due to his science-skeptic approach, Bolsonaro fiercely rejected attempts at introducing pandemic restrictions that conflicted with federal officials as well as state and local governments (Meyer 2020). What's more, the president also individually targeted governors who tried to benefit from the federal system of the country and introduce statewide protective policy measures. Health ministers who supported these governors were either fired by the president (as in the case of Luiz Henrique Mandetta) or resigned due to Bolsonaro's countermoves to reverse protective policies enacted at the state and local levels. For instance, then-Health Minister Nelson Teich resigned from office after President Bolsonaro signed an executive order to reopen gyms and beauty salons at a time when COVID-19 cases were peaking globally (Meyer 2020). Hence, under a science-skeptic populist leader, Latin America's largest country witnessed a time when a health minister could not keep his seat more than a month during the course of a global health care crisis (Londoño 2020).

The crisis cost both countries and their leaders dearly. The United States saw a US$2073 decline in GDP per capita, and Trump lost his reelection bid, even though he was seen as the likeliest to win before the pandemic started (Cox 2019). Bolsonaro likewise lost his presidential bid to Lula. Bolsonaro's Brazil also suffered from an economic breakdown before and during the pandemic. The country's GDP per capita (in US dollars) fell from $9928 in 2017 to $6796 in 2020. This economic decline on top of Bolsonaro's science-skeptic and anti-expert discourse substantially diminished the will and capacity of Brazil's national government to combat the crisis. The impact of science-skeptic discourse in the USA, where Donald Trump downplayed the scope and consequences of the infection, was that the USA had one of the highest COVID-19-related mortality rates in the world, on par with Brazil.

Brazil and the USA are federal systems. Thus, Bolsonaro and Trump had opportunity structures that differed from the those of Turkey and Israel when it came to their direct accountability for the failures of crisis response (Shvetsova et al. 2020; VanDusky-Allen et al. 2020; Adeel et al. 2020; Shvetsova et al. 2021).

Our individual location restrictions component of the PPI index consists of three components. The first component is *restricted individual mobility*: an ordinal measure that varies from 0 to 1, where 1 signifies that there is an enforced lockdown and 0 means there are no stay-at-home or curfew restrictions. The measure goes up to 0.20 if there is a curfew and no stay-at-home orders. It rises to 0.40 if there are stay-at-home orders just for specified groups, such as the elderly. It rises to 0.80 if there is a stay-at-home order for everyone.

The second component is *conditional self-isolation*. It takes a value of 1 if there is a mandatory quarantine if a person was diagnosed with or exposed to COVID or traveled. It takes a value of 0.33 if self-isolation is mandated for exposure and travel. It falls to 0 if there are no mandatory quarantines or self-isolation.

The third component is *closure of public transportation*. We include this measure here rather than closure of public gatherings since it is more about mobility than congregating. It is 0 if public transportation is open and becomes 1 if routes are closed.

In terms of individual location restrictions with all three components combined, Figure 7.2 shows Turkey and Israel scoring highest and being very close to each other. The USA's and Brazil's national scores were relatively lower. This finding is consistent with our expectations since Middle Eastern right-wing politics rely on security versus freedom when it comes to crisis response (Wheeler 2011; Hoffman 2020). Both Israel and Turkey have been embroiled in decades-long internal and external military conflicts and have political cultures that prioritize security over freedom. That's why, when Netanyahu and Erdogan restricted individual mobility, the public response and reaction were different than what an American president would face for taking the same actions. Brazil here might lie in the middle since the country experienced decades of military involvement in politics, yet they do not have the extent of conflict that the territories of Anatolia and the Levant have been exposed to.

Figure 7.3 shows that Israel's and (especially) Turkey's PPIs are mostly driven by individual location restrictions and closure of places of congregation. The fluctuation in Turkey is due to weekend partial lockdown/curfew measures. Here, the individual location restrictions also have an authoritarian tint in banning protests and political gatherings. Israeli and Turkish governments used this restriction in an effort to demobilize the opposition since both governments were in major crisis (constitutional and economic respectively). Turkey hesitates to close down places of congregation for religious and economic reasons (mosques and shopping malls), yet the government does not hesitate to restrict individual and collective freedoms of movement, mobilization, and protest. Israel took a more holistic approach on these restrictions and introduced them simultaneously within their national security crisis framework.

Our *closures of places of human congregation* measure is built on five components. The first component is a dichotomous variable that measures whether government offices are closed (2) or open (0). Second, we look at whether nonessential businesses are ordered to close down (2) or not (0). Third, we specifically code whether restaurants are forced to close down (0–2). The fourth component we use for this measure is the closure

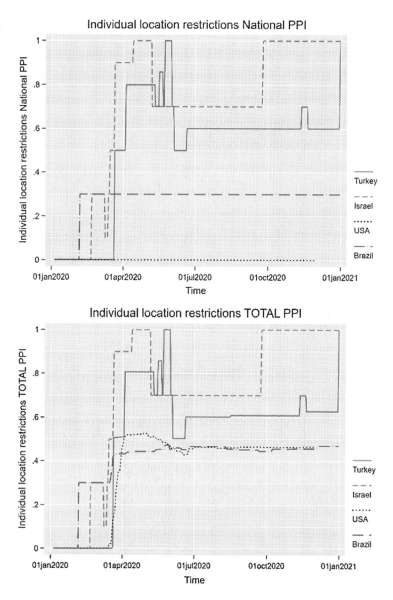

Fig. 7.2 Comparison of stringency of policies on individual location restrictions in Brazil, Israel, Turkey, and the USA, as measured by national PPI (*top*) and total PPI (*bottom*). (Source: Shvetsova et al. 2022)

7 POPULIST RESPONSES TO COVID-19: TURKEY AND ISRAEL AS CASES... 165

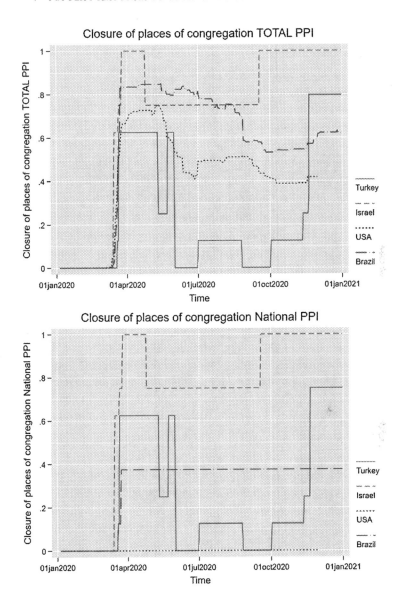

Fig. 7.3 Comparison of stringency of restrictions in places of congregation in Brazil, Israel, Turkey, and the USA, as measured by national PPI (*top*) and total PPI (*bottom*). (Source: Shvetsova et al. 2022)

of entertainment venues and stadiums (0–1). Lastly, we look at whether there is a government requirement for businesses and organizations to work from home (0–1).

In this submeasure, Israel's disproportionate response is still clear. According to the total PPI levels, the Turkish population is the least protected. Turkey eased off most of its protective measures since the government prioritized the economy over the pandemic during the summer of 2020. Further, the economic expectations from the tourism industry were also a contributing factor in Turkey's underreaction.

7.7 Conclusion

A wide array of qualitative and quantitative data presented in this chapter on populist government behavior during the COVID-19 pandemic is not uniform. Here we explored a variation of populist government that had serious implications during the first year of the pandemic: proscience and science-skeptic populism. Erdogan's and Netanyahu's governments represented proscience populism, while the Trump administration and the Bolsonaro government represented science-skeptic populism. In our findings, the Israeli and Turkish national governments responded to the COVID-19 crisis more directly, whereas the Brazilian and American administrations delegated their crisis response to federated units, further sabotaging the provincial/state-level implementation of protective measures. However, we should note that even though Erdogan's government avoided science-skeptic discourse, it relied heavily on the suppression of daily COVID-19 cases and death rates, a practice that continues to this day (World Health Organization 2022). Thus, we conclude that this variation in populist government behavior also depends on institutional arrangements and contextual pressures.

Second, we demonstrated that government behavior during the first year of the COVID-19 pandemic provides us with excellent opportunities to explore how different types of leaders react to crises and how their countries' institutional setup or contextual pressures shape their behavior. Israel and Turkey as examples of proscience populism responded to the COVID-19 crisis by taking it seriously and framing it as a familiar security crisis. Erdogan and Netanyahu attempted to use the crisis as an opportunity to reconsolidate their weakening coalitions. However, their attempts were overwhelmingly determined by the crisis and contextual pressures they faced right before and during the pandemic. On the one hand, the

7 POPULIST RESPONSES TO COVID-19: TURKEY AND ISRAEL AS CASES... 167

deep economic crisis Erdogan's government faced heavily restricted his options in implementing protective measures when they were unpopular and economically costly. On the other hand, Israel's relative prosperity during the pandemic allowed Netanyahu to overreact when it was necessary for his own and his government's survival. Nevertheless, neither Netanyahu nor Erdogan relied on a science-skeptic discourse.[10] Other populists such as Donald Trump and Jair Bolsonaro relied heavily on a science-skeptic discourse, spreading misinformation and conspiracy theories and pacifying and sabotaging the national and provincial/state-level responses to the pandemic, which cost them and their countries dearly.

Third, our findings indicate that science-skeptic populism had a negative impact on the implementation of protective policies, leading to higher levels of social and economic costs for the USA and Brazil. Trump and Bolsonaro willingly pacified the national response and sabotaged the provincial/state-level attempts. Besides these leaders' attempts, most federated units and their governments in these countries corrected their national governments' lack of response. These results support the literature that argues federalism's positive impact on the implementation of protective policies and overall protection of citizens.

We acknowledge that different factors play into how governments responded to the pandemic. Populist leadership is only one factor among many that shaped the extent and the manner in which governments responded to the pandemic. As recent literature indicates, institutional setup is one of the most important factors that played into governments' calculations and capabilities.[11] Factors such as a country's rate of urbanization and population density also likely change the speed and extent of COVID-19 spread as well as government response. In our cases, urbanization seems to be irrelevant for COVID deaths since Turkey and Brazil are the least urbanized among the four. There is also evidence from other cases that support our conclusion (see Yu et al. 2020 for China); however, other studies present mixed (González-Val and Sanz-Gracia 2022) and positive findings for urbanization's impact on COVID-19-related deaths (see Chang et al. 2022 for a macro analysis and Upadhyaya et al. 2022 for a micro analysis). Our four case studies support the idea that population density shows a positive correlation with mortality. Chang et al. (2022)

---

[10] See pp. 11–12 for more details of such exceptions.

[11] Please refer to our initial analysis and discussion on the institutional factors in this variation in the online appendix.

also found that population density aggravated the mortality rates in their cross-country analysis on 91 countries. Further research should look into how protective policies and other factors interact with each other when it comes to the extent of morbidity and mortality of the COVID-19 pandemic.

REFERENCES

Adeel AB, Catalano M, Catalano O, Gibson G, Muftuoglu E, Riggs T, Sezgin MH, Shvetsova O, Tahir N, VanDusky-Allen J, Zhao T, Zhirnov A (2020) COVID-19 policy response and the rise of the sub-national governments. Canadian Public Policy, 46(4), 565–584 https://doi.org/10.3138/cpp.2020-101.

Andone D (2020, April 17) Protests are popping up across the US over stay-at-home restrictions. CNN. https://www.cnn.com/2020/04/16/us/protests-coronavirus-stay-home-orders/index.html Accessed 5 September 2022.

Bayerlein M, Boese VA, Gates S, Kamin K, Murshed SM (2021) Populism and COVID-19: how populist governments (mis)handle the pandemic. Working Paper by Kiel Institute for the World Economy. https://www.ifw-kiel.de/fileadmin/Dateiverwaltung/IfW-Publications/-ifw/Kiel_Working_Paper/2021/KWP_2192_Bayerlein_Boese_Gates_Kamin_Murshed_/KWP_2192.pdf Accessed 5 September 2022.

BBC News (2021, May 30) Israeli opposition inch closer to deal to oust Netanyahu https://www.bbc.com/news/world-middle-east-57300769 Accessed 10 September 2022.

BBC News Turkish (2020, May 28) Mosques are opening: what are the precautions and regulations? [Originally published in Turkish "Camiler açılıyor: Hangi önlemler alındı, uyulacak kurallar neler?"] https://www.bbc.com/turkce/haberler-turkiye-52817397 Accessed 10 September 2022.

BBC News Turkish (2021, February 24) Why does the opposition criticize the AKP government, and how does the government defend itself? [Originally published in Turkish "Lebalep kongreler: Muhalefet neden eleştiriyor, AKP nasıl savunuyor?"] https://www.bbc.com/turkce/haberler-turkiye-56177899 Accessed 10 September 2022.

BBC News Turkish (2022, May 5) WHO: 2.7 times more people died in Turkey than announced [Originally published in Turkish "WHO'dan Covid-19 ölümleri hesaplaması: Türkiye'de açıklananın 2,7 katı kişi hayatını kaybetti"] https://www.bbc.com/turkce/haberler-dunya-61333377 Accessed 10 September 2022.

Boin A, Ekengren M, Rhinard M (2020) Hiding in plain sight: conceptualizing the creeping crisis. Risk, Hazards, & Crisis in Public Policy, 11(2), 116–138 https://doi.org/10.1002/rhc3.12193.

Bolukbasi M (2012) From national outlook to conservative democracy: the transformation of Islamic elites in Turkey after the February 28 process [Originally published in Turkish "Milli Görüş'ten muhafazakar demokrasiye: Türkiye'de 28 Şubat süreci sonrasi İslami elitlerin dönüşümü"], İnsan ve Toplum Bilimleri Araştırmaları Dergisi, 1(2), 166–187. https://dergipark.org.tr/tr/download/article-file/92755 Accessed 20 September 2022.

Brito R, Fonseca P (March 17, 2021) Bolsonaro opposes social distancing as Brazil sets record 90,000 COVID-19 cases. Reuters. https://www.reuters.com/article/us-health-coronavirus-brazil-cases-idUKKBN2B92ZA Accessed 5 September 2022.

Brubaker R (2021) Paradoxes of populism during the pandemic. Thesis Eleven, 164(1), 73–87 https://doi.org/10.1177/0725513620970804.

Bump P (October 6, 2020) 210,000 deaths later, Trump reverts to comparing the coronavirus to the flu. The Washington Post. https://www.washingtonpost.com/politics/2020/10/06/210000-deaths-later-trump-reverts-comparing-coronavirus-flu/ Accessed 5 September 2022.

Buncombe A (2018, May 5) Trump claims vaccines and autism are linked but his own experts vehemently disagree. Independent. https://www.independent.co.uk/news/world/americas/trump-vaccines-autism-links-anti-vaxxer-us-president-false-vaccine-a8331836.html Accessed 5 September 2022.

Cagaptay S (2020) The new sultan: Erdogan and the crisis of modern Turkey. Bloomsbury Publishing.

Castanho Silva B, Fuks M, Tamaki ER (2022) So thin it's almost invisible: populist attitudes and voting behavior in Brazil. Electoral Studies, 75(102434) 10.1016/j.electstud.2021.102434.

Cathey L (October 2, 2020) Trump, downplaying virus, has mocked wearing masks for months. ABC News. https://abcnews.go.com/Politics/trump-downplaying-virus-mocked-wearing-masks-months/story?id=73392694 Accessed 5 September 2020.

Chang D, Chang X, He Y, Tan KJK (2022) The determinants of COVID-19 morbidity and mortality across countries. Scientific Reports, 12(1): 5888, 1–17 https://doi.org/10.1038/s41598-022-09783-9.

CNN (2020a, October 2) Trump makes fun of Biden's mask-wearing habits. https://www.cnn.com/videos/politics/2020/10/02/trump-biden-masks-debate-dpx-vpx-sot.cnn Accessed 10 September 2022.

CNN (2020b, November 3) Exit Polls https://www.cnn.com/election/2020/exit-polls/president/national-results Accessed 3 September 2022.

Concoran KE, Scheitle CP, DiGregorio BD (2021) Christian nationalism and COVID-19 vaccine hesitancy and uptake. Vaccine, 39(45), 6614–6621 https://doi.org/10.1016/j.vaccine.2021.09.074.

Cox J (2019, October 15) Trump is on his way to an easy win in 2020, according to Moody's accurate election model. CNBC. https://www.cnbc.com/2019/10/15/moodys-trump-on-his-way-to-an-easy-2020-win-if-economy-holds-up.html.

Cheatham A (April 2, 2020) Skeptical Bolsonaro clashes with governors as coronavirus spreads in Brazil. Council on Foreign Relations. https://www.cfr.org/in-brief/skeptical-bolsonaro-clashes-governors-coronavirus-spreads-brazil Accessed on 5 September 2022.

Cupolo D (2020a, October 15) Erdogan demands new laws to reel in Turkish medical group. Al-Monitor. https://www.al-monitor.com/originals/2020/10/erdogan-new-laws-muzzle-turkish-medical-association.html.

Cupolo D (2020b, August 3) Turkish health officials watch for COVID-19 cases to rise after holiday. Al-Monitor. https://www.al-monitor.com/originals/2020/08/turkey-health-officials-warn-covid-rise-holiday-eid.html.

Cupolo D (2020c, October 1) Turkish Health Ministry admits to posting partial COVID-19 data. Al-Monitor. https://www.al-monitor.com/originals/2020/10/turkey-health-ministry-partial-virus-data.html.

Deane C, Parker K, Gramlich J (2021, March 5) A year of U.S. public opinion on the coronavirus pandemic. Pew Research Center. https://www.pewresearch.org/2021/03/05/a-year-of-u-s-public-opinion-on-the-coronavirus-pandemic/ Accessed 7 September 2022.

Deutsche Welle (2020, June 4) How Brazil's Evangelicals are spinning COVID-19 https://www.dw.com/en/brazil-evangelicals-preach-covid-19/a-53024007 Accessed 7 September 2022.

Dietz T (2020) Political events and public views on climate change. Climatic Change, 161, 1–8 https://link.springer.com/article/10.1007/s10584-020-02791-6

Duran AE (2017, July 1) Evolution discussion in curriculum is taken to court [Originally published in Turkish "Müfredattan çıkan evrim mahkemelik oluyor"]. Deutsche Welle. https://www.dw.com/tr/müfredattan-çıkan-evrim-mahkemelik-oluyor/a-39487990 Accessed 10 September 2022.

Enders A, Farhart C, Miller J, Uscinski J, Saunders K, Drochon H (2022) Are Republicans and Conservatives more likely to believe conspiracy theories?. Political Behavior, 1–24 https://doi.org/10.1007/s11109-022-09812-3.

Erdogan E, Semerci PU (2018, March 12) Attitudes towards Syrians in Turkey-2017. German Marshall Fund discussion on Turkish perceptions of Syrian refugees, Ankara, Turkey. https://goc.bilgi.edu.tr/media/uploads/2018/03/15/turkish-perceptions-of-syrian-refugees-20180315_Y0gYZoI.pdf Accessed 15 September 2022.

Erisen C (2022) Psychological foundations and behavioral consequences of COVID-19 conspiracy theory beliefs: the Turkish case. International Political Science Review, 01925121221084625. https://doi.org/10.1177/01925121221084625.

Firozi P (July 21, 2020). The Health 202: Trump administration resists federal mask mandate as other nations implement them. The Washington Post. https://www.washingtonpost.com/politics/2020/07/21/health-202-trump-administration-resists-federal-mask-mandate-other-nations-implement-them/ Accessed 5 September 2022.

Foa RS, Romero-Vidal X, Klassen AJ, Fuenzalida Concha J, Quednau M, Fenner LS (2022) The great reset: public opinion, populism, and the pandemic. Cambridge, United Kingdom: Centre for the Future of Democracy. https://www.bennettinstitute.cam.ac.uk/publications/great-reset/ Accessed 8 September 2022.

France24 (2020, September 28) Israel's ultra-Orthodox Jews defy Covid-19 fears during Yom Kippur https://www.france24.com/en/20200928-israel-s-ultra-orthodox-jews-defy-covid-19-fears-during-yom-kippur Accessed 10 September 2022.

Funk C, Hefferon M (2019, November 25) U.S. Public Views on Climate and Energy. Pew Research Center. https://www.pewresearch.org/science/2019/11/25/u-s-public-views-on-climate-and-energy/ Accessed 8 September 2022.

Funk C (2020, February 12) Key findings about Americans' confidence in science and their views on scientists' role in society. Pew Research Center. https://www.pewresearch.org/fact-tank/2020/02/12/key-findings-about-americans-confidence-in-science-and-their-views-on-scientists-role-in-society/ Accessed 8 September 2022.

Funk C, Tyson A (2020, June 3) Partisan differences over the pandemic response are growing. Pew Research Center. https://www.pewresearch.org/science/2020/06/03/partisan-differences-over-the-pandemic-response-are-growing/ Accessed 8 September 2022.

Gesser-Edelsburg A, Hijazi R (2020) When politics meets pandemic: How Prime Minister Netanyahu and a small team communicated health and risk information to the Israeli public during the early stages of COVID-19. *Risk Management and Healthcare Policy, 13*, 2985 https://doi.org/10.2147/RMHP.S280952

González-Val R, Sanz-Gracia F (2022) Urbanization and COVID-19 incidence: a cross-country investigation. Papers in Regional Science, 101(2), 399–415 https://doi.org/10.1111/pirs.12647.

Hoffman A (2020) The securitization of the coronavirus crisis in the Middle East. The COVID-19 pandemic in the Middle East and North Africa, 10. https://pomeps.org/the-securitization-of-the-coronavirus-crisis-in-the-middle-east Accessed 8 September 2022.

Human Rights Watch (April 10, 2020) Brazil: Bolsonaro sabotages anti-Covid-19 efforts. https://www.hrw.org/news/2020/04/10/brazil-bolsonaro-sabotages-anti-covid-19-efforts Accessed 5 September 2022.

Huber RA (2020) The role of populist attitudes in explaining climate change skepticism and support for environmental protection. Environmental Politics, 29(6), 959–982 https://doi.org/10.1080/09644016.2019.1708186.

Kavakli KC (2020) Did populist leaders respond to the COVID-19 pandemic more slowly? Evidence from a global sample. (Working Paper). https://kerimcan81.files.wordpress.com/2020/06/covidpop-main-2020-06-18.pdf Accessed 5 September 2022.

Kisa S, Kisa A (2020) Under-reporting of COVID-19 cases in Turkey. The International Journal of Health Planning and Management, 35(5), 1009–1013 https://doi.org/10.1002/hpm.3031.

Laebens MG, Ozturk A (2021) Partisanship and autocratization: polarization, power asymmetry, and partisan social identities in Turkey. Comparative Political Studies, 54(2), 245–279 https://doi.org/10.1177/0010414020926199.

Laebens MG, Ozturk A (2022) The Erdogan government's response to the COVID-19 pandemic: performance and actuality in an authoritarian context. Government and Opposition, 1–18 https://doi.org/10.1017/gov.2022.16.

Laudicina P (2021, May 12) Can populism survive the pandemic? Forbes. https://www.forbes.com/sites/paullaudicina/2021/05/12/can-populism-survive-the-pandemic/?sh=2587fc1b6d0a.

Londoño E (2020, May 15) Another health minister in Brazil exits amid chaotic coronavirus response. The New York Times. https://www.nytimes.com/2020/05/15/world/americas/brazil-health-minister-bolsonaro.html Accessed 5 September 2022.

Maor M, Sulitzeanu-Kenan R, Chinitz D (2020) When COVID-19, constitutional crisis, and political deadlock meet: the Israeli case from a disproportionate policy perspective. Policy and Society, 39(3), 442–457 https://academic.oup.com/policyandsociety/article/39/3/442/6407894.

Meyer B (2020, August 17) Pandemic populism: an analysis of populist leaders' responses to COVID-19. https://institute.global/policy/pandemic-populism-analysis-populist-leaders-responses-covid-19 Accessed 5 August 2022.

Miller ME (2015, September 17) The GOP's 'dangerous' debate on vaccines and autism. The Washington Post. https://www.washingtonpost.com/news/morning-mix/wp/2015/09/17/the-gops-dangerous-debate-on-vaccines-and-autism/ Accessed 5 September 2022.

Miller JD, Scott EC, Ackerman MS, Laspra B, Branch G, Polino C, Huffaker JS (2022) Public acceptance of evolution in the United States, 1985–2020. Public Understanding of Science, 31(2), 223–238 https://doi.org/10.1177/09636625211035919.

Mitchell TG (2015) Likud leaders: the lives and careers of Menahem Begin, Yitzhak Shamir, Benjamin Netanyahu and Ariel Sharon. McFarland.

Mitchell A, Jurkowitz M, Oliphant JB, Shearer E (2021, February 22) Republicans' views on COVID-19 shifted over course of 2020; Democrats' hardly budged. Pew Research Center. https://www.pewresearch.org/journalism/2021/02/22/republicans-views-on-covid-19-shifted-over-course-of-2020-democrats-hardly-budged/ Accessed 8 September 2022.

Mounk Y (2021, April 26) How populism has proven lethal in this pandemic. Council on Foreign Relations (Originally published at *Folha de S.Paulo*). https://www.cfr.org/article/how-populism-has-proven-lethal-pandemic Accessed 5 September 2022.

Mudde C (2004) The populist zeitgeist. Government and Opposition, 39(4), 541–563 https://doi.org/10.1111/j.1477-7053.2004.00135.x.

Mudde C (2017) An ideational approach. In C. R. Kaltwasser, P. Taggart, P. Ochoa Espejo, & P. Ostiguy (Eds.), The Oxford handbook of populism. (1st ed., pp. 27–47). Oxford University Press. https://doi.org/10.1093/oxfordhb/9780198803560.013.1.

Naushirvanov T, Rosenberg D, Sawyer P, Seyis D (2022) "How populists fueled polarization and failed their response to Covid-19: an empirical analysis". Forthcoming in Frontiers in Political Science. https://doi.org/10.3389/fpos.2022.948137.

Neiwert D (2017) Alt-America: the rise of the radical right in the age of Trump. Verso Books.

O'Brien TL, Noy S (2020) Political identity and confidence in science and religion in the United States. Sociology of Religion, 81(4), 439–461 https://doi.org/10.1093/socrel/sraa024.

Pardhan S, Drydakis N (2021) Associating the change in new COVID-19 cases to GDP per capita in 38 European countries in the first wave of the pandemic. Frontiers in Public Health, 8, 582140 https://doi.org/10.3389/fpubh.2020.582140.

Pazzanese C (October 27, 2020). Calculating possible fallout of Trump's dismissal of face masks. The Harvard Gazette. https://news.harvard.edu/gazette/story/2020/10/possible-fallout-from-trumps-dismissal-of-face-masks/ Accessed September 2022.

Peleg I (2019) The Likud under Benjamin Netanyahu: readjusting revisionism to the 21st century. In R. O. Friedman (Ed.), Israel Under Netanyahu (pp. 11–32). Routledge.

Perez M (April 11, 2020) Report: Trump ignored pleas to put social distancing practices in place, warnings of a pandemic. Forbes. https://www.forbes.com/sites/mattperez/2020/04/11/report-trump-ignored-pleas-to-put-social-distancing-practices-in-place-warnings-of-a-pandemic/?sh=6815b524751f Accessed 5 September 2022.

Phillips T (2020a, March 23) Brazil's Jair Bolsonaro says coronavirus crisis is a media trick. The Guardian. https://www.theguardian.com/world/2020/mar/23/brazils-jair-bolsonaro-says-coronavirus-crisis-is-a-media-trick Accessed 5 September 2022.

Phillips T (2020b, July 8) Brazil: Bolsonaro reportedly uses homophobic slur to mock masks. The Guardian. https://www.theguardian.com/world/2020/jul/08/bolsonaro-masks-slur-brazil-coronavirus Accessed 5 September 2022.

Ray E (March 7, 2022) Truckers protesting Covid mandates are amassing outside the capital. The New York Times. https://www.nytimes.com/live/2022/03/05/world/covid-19-tests-cases-vaccine#trucker-convoy-washington-protest Accessed 5 September 2022.

Ramsay S (June 21, 2021) COVID-19: Bolsonaro doesn't believe in social distancing, masks or vaccines. That wasn't lost on those protesting. Sky News. https://news.sky.com/story/covid-19-in-brazil-the-fact-500-000-have-died-and-the-country-isnt-in-lockdown-is-too-much-for-some-to-take-12336762 Accessed 5 September 2022.

Renno LR (2020) The Bolsonaro voter: issue positions and vote choice in the 2018 Brazilian presidential elections. Latin American Politics and Society, 62(4), 1–23 https://doi.org/10.1017/lap.2020.13.

Rutjens BT, Sengupta N, Van Der Lee R, Van Koningsbruggen GM, Martens JP, Rabelo A, Sutton RM (2022) Science skepticism across 24 countries. Social Psychological and Personality Science, 13(1), 102–117 https://doi.org/10.1177/19485506211001329.

Selcuki C (2021, October 26) How do the low-income AKP voters get poorer but not flee? Yetkin Report. https://yetkinreport.com/en/2021/10/26/how-do-the-low-income-akp-voters-get-poorer-but-not-flee/ Accessed 10 September 2022.

Seyis D (2021, March 20) Populists' health care policies during the COVID-19 pandemic [Published originally in Turkish: "COVID-19 sürecinde popülistlerin sağlık politikaları"]. Istanbul Political Research Institute. https://www.istanpol.org/post-covid-19-surecinde-pop-listlerin-saglik-politikalar Accessed 2 September 2022.

Shvetsova O, Zhirnov A, VanDusky-Allen J, Adeel AB, Catalano M, Catalano O, Giannelli F, Muftuoglu E, Riggs T, Sezgin MH, Tahir N, Zhao T (2020) Institutional origins of protective COVID-19 public health policy responses: informational and authority redundancies and policy stringency. Journal of Political Institutions and Political Economy, 1(4), 585–613 https://doi.org/10.1561/113.00000023

Shvetsova O, VanDusky-Allen J, Zhirnov A, Adeel AB, Catalano M, Catalano O, Giannelli F, Muftuoglu E, Rosenberg D, Sezgin MH, Zhao T (2021) Federal institutions and strategic policy responses to COVID-19 pandemic. Frontiers in Political Science. 3(631363) https://doi.org/10.3389/fpos.2021.631363.

Shvetsova O, Zhirnov A, Adeel AB, Bayar MC, Bayrali OG, Catalano M, Catalano O, Chu H, Giannelli F, Muftuoglu E, Rosenberg D, Seyis D, Skopyk B, VanDusky-Allen J, Zhao T (2022) Protective policy index (PPI) global dataset of origins and stringency of COVID 19 mitigation policies. Scientific Data, 9, 319 https://doi.org/10.1038/s41597-022-01437-9.

Staerklé C, Cavallaro M, Cortijos-Bernabeu A, Bonny S (2022) Common sense as a political weapon: populism, science skepticism, and global crisis-solving motivations. Political Psychology, 43(5), 913–929 https://doi.org/10.1111/pops.12823.

Staff T (2018, 30 August) Israeli schools largely avoid teaching evolution. The Times of Israel. https://www.timesofisrael.com/israeli-schools-largely-avoid-teaching-evolution-report/ Accessed 10 September 2022.

Stewart E (2020, August 7) Anti-maskers explain themselves. Vox. https://www.vox.com/the-goods/2020/8/7/21357400/anti-mask-protest-rallies-donald-trump-covid-19 Accessed 8 September 2022.

Upadhyaya A, Koirala S, Ressler R, Upadhyaya K (2022) Factors affecting COVID-19 mortality: an exploratory study. Journal of Health Research, 36(1), 166–175 https://doi.org/10.1108/JHR-09-2020-0448.

VanDusky-Allen J, Shvetsova O, Zhirnov A (2020, June 17) Brazilian federalism and state level policy responses to the COVID-19 pandemic. Blue Review. https://www.boisestate.edu/bluereview/brazilian-federalism/ Accessed 3 August 2022.

Veldman RG (2019) The gospel of climate skepticism. Why Evangelical Christians oppose action on climate change. University of California Press.

Victor D, Serviss L, Paybarah A (October 2, 2020) In his own words, Trump on the coronavirus and masks. The New York Times. https://www.nytimes.com/2020/10/02/us/politics/donald-trump-masks.html Accessed 5 September 2022.

Waitzberg R, Davidovitch N, Leibner G, Penn N, Brammli-Greenberg S (2020) Israel's response to the COVID-19 pandemic: tailoring measures for vulnerable cultural minority populations. International Journal for Equity in Health, 19(71) 10.1186/s12939-020-01191-7.

Wheeler D (2011) Freedom from want, and freedom from fear: a human security approach to a new Middle East?. Journal of Human Security, 7(1), 37–52 https://doi.org/10.3316/JHS0701037.

Wolfe D, Dale D (October 31, 2020) 'It's going to disappear': A timeline of Trump's claims that Covid-19 will vanish. CNN. https://www.cnn.com/interactive/2020/10/politics/covid-disappearing-trump-comment-tracker/ Accessed 5 September 2022.

World Bank (2022) GDP Per Capita (US$) World Bank national accounts data, and OECD National Accounts data files. https://data.worldbank.org/indicator/NY.GDP.MKTP.CD?end=2020&locations=US-TR-IL-BR&start=2016 Accessed 11 September 2022.

World Health Organization (2022) Global excess deaths associated with COVID-19 (modelled estimates). https://www.who.int/data/sets/global-excess-deaths-associated-with-covid-19-modelled-estimates Accessed 10 September 2022.

Yu F, Du L, Ojcius DM, Pan C, Jiang S (2020) Measures for diagnosing and treating infections by a novel coronavirus responsible for a pneumonia outbreak originating in Wuhan, China. Microbes Infect, 22(2), 74–79 https://doi.org/10.1016/j.micinf.2020.01.003

Zimmer C (2020, October 1) Fauci pushes back against Trump for misrepresenting his stance on masks. The New York Times. https://www.nytimes.com/2020/10/01/world/fauci-pushes-back-against-trump-for-misrepresenting-his-stance-on-masks.html Accessed 10 September 2022.

CHAPTER 8

The Visegrad Populist Leaders' Responses to COVID-19 Pandemic

Hyoungrohk Chu

8.1 Introduction

The Visegrad countries, the Czech Republic, Hungary, Poland, and Slovakia,[1] have a number of things in common. First, they are all geographically located in Central Europe. Second, following the collapse of the Soviet Union, these postcommunist countries made a successful transition to capitalism and liberal democracy and recently joined the European Union. Third, their healthcare policies have continued to be influenced by

---

[1] The term *Visegrad group/countries* (or simply V4) refers to a political alliance of Czechia, Hungary, Poland, and Slovakia within the EU. Historically, these four countries share a lot of political, socioeconomic, cultural, and religious traditions. Against this backdrop, the V4 have worked together in many aspects, such as the economy, foreign policy, defense, energy, and so on (Visegrad Group 2022). For further information, please visit this website: https://www.visegradgroup.eu/about.

H. Chu (✉)
Department of Political Science, Binghamton University,
Binghamton, NY, USA
e-mail: hchu13@binghamton.edu

© The Author(s), under exclusive license to Springer Nature Switzerland AG 2023
O. Shvetsova (ed.), *Government Responses to the COVID-19 Pandemic*, https://doi.org/10.1007/978-3-031-30844-4_8

177

178   H. CHU

the Semashko-style healthcare system (Heinrich 2022).[2] Lastly, in relation to this volume, when the pandemic broke out in 2020, all four Visegrad countries (V4) had populists heading the executive branch of government. This coincidence has created a natural experiment that makes it possible to compare their approaches to pandemic management. Here is one intriguing result. The V4 seemed to manage the pandemic well in spring 2020 but ended up failing in fall 2020. This pattern is the opposite of these countries' West European EU counterparts.[3] The puzzle is what caused the reversal in the V4. This chapter tries to shed new light on the political origins of this reversal.

This essay argues that the Visegrad leaders in the first wave of the pandemic had a comparative advantage in imposing the necessary nonmedical interventions (NMIs) because of a combination of path-dependent institutional and post-Soviet legacy variables. Specifically, the already dominant executives driven by an erosion of democracy showed tentative proscience attitudes for pandemic mitigation and, thus, made good use of highly centralized governance of public health inherited from the Semashko-style healthcare systems and planned economies. This advantage enabled the V4 incumbents to capitalize politically on their handling of the initial stage of the pandemic.

In the fall of 2020, however, their pandemic responses were no longer timely or sufficient. My explanation for the reversal of the V4 executives' pandemic strategies is that public confidence and the economic outlook took a bad turn. Initially, the V4 had a high level of public confidence, optimistic economic prospects, and even epidemiological luck, meaning that the virus arrived late in the V4 territories and spread to the region relatively slowly. Combined, these features led to the popular perception of government success in doing what other countries in Europe had failed to do – namely, to protect their public. However, the V4's policy strategies changed in the fall, despite the favorable institutional legacies, because demand-side factors reversed such that prompt and strict policies were no

---

[2] Inherited from the former Soviet Union's socialist healthcare system, the term *Semashko-style healthcare system* means a nationalized (funded by the national budget), centralized, unified healthcare system that is free of charge and equal for every citizen. Nowadays, its major features and problems include excessive inpatient capacity (e.g., the number of hospital beds per 1000 people), weak health-workforce policy, the gap between urban and rural areas, and low quality of care, for example (Sagan et al. 2022, p. 446; Sheiman et al. 2018).

[3] In this chapter, Western European comparisons include Austria, Belgium, France, Germany, Ireland, Netherlands, and the United Kingdom.

longer low-cost to incumbents in electoral terms. Public attitudes were changed by the eventual massive spread of COVID-19 and the signs of mounting economic costs of pandemic mitigation, which called into question the effectiveness of the governments' prior decisions. As the expected electoral costs of incumbents' stringent protections escalated, the place science occupied in their decisions became diminished. Thus, the V4 populist leaders' actions in the second wave were consistent with purely political calculations, which demonstrates that both proscience attitudes and the will to put into place protective NMIs in the first wave were based on their instrumental reelection value.

8.2 Theory: What Enabled the V4's Quick and Strong NMI Policies?

Before investigating the factors in the decision-making around the pandemic, we need to first conceptualize populism. Following Mudde's ideational approach, populism includes two primary elements. The first is the Manichean antagonistic division of the pure people versus the corrupt elite. The second is that populist politicians should represent the general will in the name of popular sovereignty, because mainstream politics has escaped from popular control (Mudde 2004). Once these two criteria are fulfilled, populism as a thin ideology is malleable and can blend with any host ideology. Accordingly, the way populism works in the real world is fairly chameleonic (Taggart 2004). While many populists are ideologically on the far right or far left of the political spectrum, some are situated around the center or "valence" (the latter means that it is not easy to put them on the traditional left-right political spectrum). Viktor Orban (Fidsez, Hungary) and Mateusz Morawiecki (PiS, Poland) are normally categorized as far-right populists, whereas Andrej Babis (ANO, Czech Republic) and Igor Matovic (OĽANO, Slovakia) are regarded as valence populist leaders (Zulianello 2020, Table 8.1).[4]

[4] For further details on populist party classification, please refer to PopuList (Rooduijn et al. 2019) and Global Party Survey (Norris 2020). There is general agreement among scholars that Fidsez and PiS are far-right or radical-right populist parties, but ANO and OĽANO might be tricky. Nevertheless, Zulianello (2020) explicitly classifies them as valence populist parties. In line with this, Bustikova and Babos (2020) illustrate that both parties adopt technocratic populism, which is distinct from right-wing or left-wing populism. First, they do not stick to a traditional (left-right) ideological spectrum. Second, they "have flexible and opportunistic policy platforms that respond to shifts in public moods, social media impulses, and extensive internal polling" (Bustikova and Babos 2020, p. 498).

180   H. CHU

Table 8.1 A theoretical framework for V4's pandemic handling in 2020

Factor	Institution		Popular support	
	Executive capacity (autonomy)	Healthcare organization	Public confidence	Economic outlook
Wave				
Spring (1st)	Strong (high)	Centralized and public health orientation	High↑	Rosy↑
Fall (2nd)	Strong (high)	Centralized and public health orientation	Low↓	Gloomy↓

8.2.1 Institutions I: Strong Executive Capacity and Autonomy

The V4 all shares two political features. Not only is the form of government a unitary parliamentary system, but this region has also experienced democratic backsliding from liberal democracy to electoral democracy or electoral autocracy throughout the 2010s. Power has become concentrated around the central government, and the role of liberal mediating institutions has become weaker. Why is this trend important here? As a means to eclipse the V4's weak healthcare system (e.g., chronic underfunding, exodus of skilled health-sector workforce, low quality of care)[5], it is very likely that each government wanted to establish quick and harsh preventive measures to stop the spread of COVID-19 in the early phase. At this point, the V4's highly centralized policymaking structure is a big asset to its leaders in power, which results from the ongoing democratic erosion in combination with a post-planned-economy legacy. In addition to this, populist leaders in times of crisis are more likely than nonpopulist leaders to aggrandize the executive under the pretext of enhancing its capacity in response to the crisis. The sudden pandemic outbreak is surely a crisis, but it is also a good chance for populist leaders to prove their political competence, advertise their governing skills, and concentrate power in the executive again, especially when we see no alternative but to depend on the government's NMIs. As a result, populist leaders are

[5] Please see "Health Indicator" in Table 8.2. The EU average in each health index is as follows (Sagan et al. 2022, p. 447): health spending as a share of GDP (9.9%); practicing doctors per 1000 people (3.6); practicing nurses per 1000 people (8.4); hospital beds per 1000 people (5.1). The V4's superior health indicator is only the inpatient capacity, that is, the number of hospital beds per 1000 people. The V4's scores in this indicator are all above the EU average (5.1): Czechia (6.9), Hungary (7.0), Poland (6.6), Slovakia (5.8).

motivated enough to handle the pandemic well, so the V4's initial responses will be likely propelled by the central government, that is, the head of the executive. Last but not least, the way governing coalitions are constructed is worth mentioning. If the ruling government is a majority coalition, this parliamentary setting would be institutionally advantageous for the prime minister in that the coalition could quite easily propose a bill the executive hoped to enact. In other words, a majority ruling coalition in a unitary parliamentary system has few institutional barriers in parliament that could legitimately impede executive-driven policymaking efforts. All in all, this chapter asserts that the V4 had strong executive capacity and autonomy so that its populist leaders in the face of a new threat were incentivized to take advantage of such institutional advantages to impose strict measures swiftly.

8.2.2 Institutions II: Public Health Orientation Toward Effective Epidemic Management

Based on Mudde's ideational conceptualization, several studies have shown that populist governments tended to respond to COVID-19 less effectively than nonpopulist ones (Bayerlein 2021; Kavakli 2020; Mckee 2021). They all contend that populist leaders were less likely to take the pandemic seriously owing to their skepticism toward science, experts, elites, and mediating institutions between people and the elites. For this reason, populist responses were slower and less stringent than nonpopulist ones. This was indeed true for Brazil, the United Kingdom, and the United States. Not only did leaders initially downplay the impact of a new virus, thus biasing the public against what scientists, health experts, and elite politicians were suggesting, but they also bypassed and terminated the institutions created by the professional establishment: Donald Trump wound up the Predict project, an early warning program about potential pandemics, three months prior to the coronavirus outbreak (Milman 2020). Boris Johnson abolished the cabinet pandemic committee, Threats, Hazards, Resilience, and Contingency Committee (THRCC), six months before outbreak (Walters 2020). Jair Bolsonaro described the COVID-19 crisis as a media trick by his political opponents and the established press (Phillips 2020). As a result, not only were they ill-prepared for a new virus when the first case was detected, but their skepticism about science aggravated the situation.

182   H. CHU

Meyer (2020), however, finds that it is not true that populist leaders did not comply with scientific advice. In fact, twelve out of seventeen populists analyzed in Meyer's study followed scientific suggestions in the initial stage of the pandemic. Moreover, as pointed out by Boot (2020) and Mudde (2020), there was no such thing as a single coherent populist response. If anything, the cases of Brazil, the UK, and the USA should not be overly generalized. In point of fact, the V4 leaders in the first wave can serve as prime examples of science-friendly populists – although their pro-science attitudes were contingent – in that their spring NMI policies were made according to scientific recommendations. The question is how the V4 leaders were proactively able to take a science-friendly quick step to prevent the spread of the virus, as opposed to the three aforementioned populist leaders and Western European leaders in government. Were there any favorable institutional backgrounds behind this?

It was the legacy of the V4's healthcare systems that helped leaders make scientifically correct (swift and stringent) decisions in the first wave. The V4 executives, when faced with a new pandemic, presided over the state-run Semashko-style health care system, which by design had an effective infectious disease and epidemic prevention and management orientation. Monopolized by the state and bureaucratically centralized, this system led to the establishment of extensive epidemiological monitoring networks and substantial epidemic preventive measures. The V4's excessive bed capacity, for example, originated from the assumption that infectious cases should be isolated from the society and well treated in hospitals. In a nutshell, the V4's healthcare systems were intended to be conducive to public health and social hygiene for every citizen of the country (Heinrich 2022; Manaev 2021; World Health Organization 1998). In actuality, notwithstanding major fundamental deficiencies in dealing with noninfectious diseases, they were at least able to "satisfy the early demands for better health care by staving off infections, epidemics, famines, and terribly unsanitary conditions" (Schecter 1992, p. 210). Not only did this historical healthcare legacy offer the executive a ready-made game plan for the pandemic, but it also prepared the public to see pandemic policies as a natural task of the government-owned healthcare system. Supported by both the supply side (institutional level) and demand side (mass level), the V4 executives were thereby legitimately granted the capacity to adopt the NMIs quickly and strictly.

8.2.3 Popular Support: High Level of Public Confidence and Rosy Economic Forecast

The demand for policies, from a politician's point of view, is well reflected in public opinion. Politicians are wary of acquiring a bad reputation, losing popularity, and eventually losing reelection, and for these reasons they are averse to making policies that do not have popular support. In this respect, the V4's populist politicians acted just like any other politicians. Indeed, one article demonstrates that "an excessive responsiveness to majoritarian preferences" is a "distinguishing feature of any type of populist policies" (Bartha et al. 2020, p. 71). Another article further claims that "populism as a ruling power tends to give life to governments that stretch the democratic rules toward an extreme majoritarianism" (Urbinati 2017, p. 571). Inevitably, populist leaders in power pay close attention to citizens' majoritarian opinions.

It is true for any election-minded politician that if the degree of public confidence is high, then she has no constraint on taking quick and strong actions. By contrast, if its degree is low and she becomes less popular, she has no choice but to lift stringent measures. In light of Heller et al. (2023), established parties with strong voter linkages are partially insulated from this problem, because their supporters maintain confidence in them despite some downturns. Populist leaders in government are, however, extremely sensitive to the swings in public sentiment and cannot afford to preside over any downturns; a bleak economy is a heavy political burden to them, since many people blame the government and its policies for their economic struggles. In the same vein, populist politicians do not have the leverage to reimpose the strict measures that were previously eased and discredited, since their popular support is linked only to successful performance, not to their long-term history with their core supporters. In sum, the V4's swift and strict policies in the first stage of the pandemic were contingent on the mass-level support coming from a high level of public confidence in government and its prevention measures and positive economic outlook.

8.3 Narrative I: How Did the V4 Accomplish Relative Success in Spring?

The V4's stringent NMI policies were relatively low-cost in electoral terms to adopt in the initial phase of COVID-19. Thanks to the increasing executive autonomy and public health orientation embedded in the health sector, these harsh policies were put in place faster in the V4 than in Western Europe. To be more specific, as shown in Figure 8.1, it is generally observed that the stringency index on the *y*-axis between the far-left

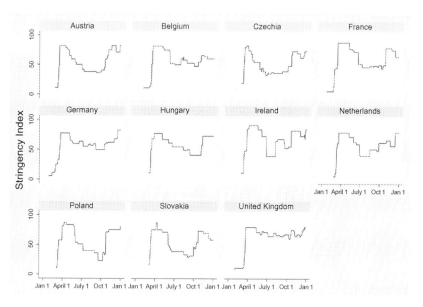

Fig. 8.1 Level of government protective policies (2020). (Source: Oxford Coronavirus Government Response Tracker (OxCGRT) (2022). Note: The Stringency Index (SI), the mean score of the following pandemic-relevant policy areas, is computed on a daily basis and thus points to how strict a set of COVID-19 nonpharmaceutical policies are: school closures, workplace closures, cancellation of public events, restriction on public gatherings, closures of public transport, stay-at-home requirements, public information campaigns, restrictions on internal movement, and international travel controls. A high SI score does not always suggest that a certain government's pandemic responses are excellent, but we can estimate whether their policy stringency is timely and sufficient especially in the absence of vaccination in 2020)

starting point (i.e., the least strict first measures during the first wave) and the first peak (i.e., the strictest measures during the first wave) increased more rapidly for a shorter period of time (i.e., shorter left tails and/or fewer stairs from the starting point to the first peak on the x-axis) in the V4 than in Western Europe. Simply put, the NMIs' stringency level skyrocketed in the V4 in a relatively shorter amount of time as compared to Western Europe. Conversely, it took longer for Western European governments to introduce the most stringent measures after the first measures. The fact that there were longer left tails and/or more stairs between the far-left starting point and the first peak simply means that Western European countries took the strongest actions only after much delay.

8.3.1 Institutions I: Executive Aggrandizement and State of Emergency

Some indicators tell us whether the V4 have strong executive capacity and autonomy. First of all, a few articles using the V-Dem index (Lindberg 2018; Gidengil et al. 2022, p. 18) clearly show that the V4's democracy has been in retreat over the past decade, that is, from liberal democracy to electoral democracy or electoral autocracy.[6] Executive aggrandizement is a typical symptom of democratic backsliding, indicating that the power of the executive and its leader becomes less restrained by the two other branches. As horizontal accountability weakens, the scope and capacity of the executive power expands in the end. Moreover, Guasti (2021) reveals that all V4 populist leaders have continued to attempt to undermine democratic accountability in the wake of the pandemic, implying that it was a good opportunity for them to rationalize executive aggrandizement in the name of protection of the people ("us") from a new threat. In turn, the V4 leaders took the lead in the pandemic policymaking procedures. As Sagan and her colleagues (2022, pp. 448–449) elucidate, the V4's offices of prime minister played a leading role in coordinating several crisis management bodies within the executive (see Table 8.2 in Sagan et al. 2022) and introducing national-level pandemic policies in the early phase of COVID-19 outbreak. This central government-led policy tendency is empirically buttressed by the Protective Policy Index (PPI), where data are documented "at subnational and national level on the daily level of stringency of public health policies by level of government overall" (Shvetsova

---

[6] Also, please refer to "Political regime (Freedom House & V-Dem Institute)" in Table 8.2.

186   H. CHU

Table 8.2 Economic/health/political indicators in the Visegrad Group

Indicator	Czechia	Hungary	Poland	Slovakia
Economic Indicator				
GDP per capita (current US $)	23,664.8	16,783.0	15,699.9	19,385.5
HDI (ranking)	0.900 (27th)	0.854 (40th)	0.880 (35th)	0.860 (39th)
Employment in agriculture (%)	2.7	4.7	9.1	2.8
Employment in industry (%)	37.3	32.1	32.1	36.1
Employment in services (%)	60.1	63.2	58.7	61.1
Internet usage (%)	80.9	80.4	80.4	82.9
Health Indicator				
Health spending as a share of GDP(%)	7.1	7.4	6.5	7.1
Practicing doctors per 1000 people	3.7	3.2	2.4	3.5
Practicing nurses per 1000 people	8.1	6.4	5.1	5.7
Hospital beds per 1000 people	6.9	7.0	6.6	5.8
Political Indicator				
Political regime (Freedom House & V-Dem Institute)	Free and electoral democracy	Partly free and electoral autocracy	Partly free and electoral democracy	Free and electoral democracy
Forms of government	Unitary and parliamentary	Unitary and parliamentary	Unitary and parliamentary	Unitary and parliamentary
Parties in government (2020)	Minority coalition	Supermajority coalition	Majority coalition	Majority coalition

Note: Economic indicators are from World Bank (2019a, b, c, d, e) and UNDP (2020). Health ones are from OECD and Sagan et al. (2022). Political ones are from Freedom House (2019), V-Dem Institute (2019), PARLINE (2018), and each country's official government website. These indicators refer mostly to 2019, but a few of them are for 2018 or 2020

et al. 2022, p. 1). This PPI dataset confirms that the V4's NMI policies were announced mostly at the national (central government) level.[7]

Another example is a state of emergency or its corresponding state of epidemic (Poland). It took less time for the Visegrad group to enforce it

---

[7] For more details about how the PPI and its subcategories are constructed, please refer to this volume's Chap. 1 and Appendix A. Further, if you want to identify at what level the V4's public health policies were announced, please go to the following website and look at the column "level" in the sheet "Check Consistency": https://github.com/COVID-policy-response-lab/PPI-data/tree/main/prelim

upon the arrival of the first case: Czechia 11 days, Hungary 7 days, Poland 10 days, and Slovakia 6 days. Meanwhile, many Western European countries did not even declare a state of emergency, had no constitutional emergency law applicable to COVID-19, or postponed its declaration (e.g., 22 days in Austria). How did the V4 declare it so quickly? First, as explained earlier, the V4 developed a highly centralized power structure or governance. Second, not only did the constitution applicable to COVID-19 exist, but the parliament's overall support enabled populist leaders to easily implement a severe state-of-emergency law nationwide. In particular, the case of Czechia is worth mentioning. Although its governing formation was a minority coalition at the time, "there was also nearly unanimous political support for the government's general anti-virus measures when they were introduced in March. No visible or substantial criticism from the opposition was formulated in this period" (Cisar and Kubat 2021, p. 111). How about the three other countries? As they all had a (super) majority coalition (e.g., two-thirds majority of Fidsez in Hungarian parliament) in spring 2020, there were few institutional obstacles in parliament that could have prevented the executive-driven strict measures, including state of emergency and national lockdown.

8.3.2 Institutions II: Public Health Orientation and Tentative Proscience Attitudes

Research has documented that the V4 populist leaders established national response teams, coordinated with them, consulted with public health experts and epidemiologists, and reflected their scientific recommendations in the first wave's pandemic policymaking procedures (Bene and Boda 2021, pp. 98–100; Cisar and Kubat 2021, p. 111; Sagan et al. 2022, pp. 448–450). This indicates that the V4 executives proactively presided over their health care systems, which had been historically keen on infectious disease management, and that they had proscience attitudes in terms of the COVID-19 NMIs. Indeed, they all took the pandemic seriously (Meyer 2020) and gave top priority to the public health sector in spring 2020. Consequently, the V4 leaders' coordination with expert advisory groups raised an awareness of the severity of the unknown virus and the necessity of the containment strategy in the early stage of the pandemic. All V4 leaders had barely any doubt about the role of science per se in lessening the spread of the disease. Here, epidemiological luck was an extra bonus, since those with a public health orientation and proscience

188 H. CHU

attitudes were given more preparation time compared to Western Europe[8] and were willing to analyze why neighboring countries were in chaos. They were thus advised to enforce stringent measures more quickly than, for example, Austria and Germany did (Guasti 2020, p. 51).

If this is the case, did the V4 populists truly believe in science? It is true that the V4's prompt and stringent protection measures in spring were ascribed to the populist leaders' tentatively giving top priority to the healthcare sector and their provisional support for science. However, they did not heed scientific warnings over the summer. In that sense, it can be said that science was instrumental to populist leaders in government. One remaining question is why they gave up their proscience attitudes in the fall. Here, note again that the basic characteristic of a populist politician is prioritizing popular majority support. When many people endorsed their policies, meaning the electoral costs were relatively low, populists were motivated to put infectious disease prevention first and abide by experts' scientific advice. However, when electoral costs increased, science, never the number one priority, was no longer followed. To put it another way, public health policies were subordinated to political and/or economic considerations.

8.3.3 Popular Support: High Level of Public Confidence and Promising Economic Outlook

The unprecedented health crisis led people to believe that the government should actively try to do something for them. In the absence of vaccination, the legacy of the Semashko-style healthcare system further encouraged them to rely upon the government's proactive NMIs. Against this backdrop, the extent of public confidence in government and its prevention measures was constantly above 50% in the first wave (European National Panels 2020, see the Government Confidence Index March 18, 2020–April 22, 2020). It may have been part of a rally-round-the-flag effect, but regardless, this level of support made it possible for the government to take immediate and decisive actions and hence contain the virus effectively. Also, the same survey tells us that many people were very

---

[8] The specific arrival dates of the first confirmed cases were as follows: Czech Republic: March 1; Hungary: March 4; Poland: March 4; and Slovakia: March 6 versus Austria: February 25; Belgium: February 4; France: January 24; Germany: January 27; Ireland: February 29; the Netherlands: February 27: and the UK: January 31.

concerned about this unknown disease; the degree of panic was around 65% to 75% during the same period (March 18, 2020–April 22, 2020). In addition, the V4's economies were performing very well prior to the outbreak of COVID-19, so that the economic outlook for 2020 was initially optimistic (Bene and Boda 2021, p. 88; Bukowski 2021; Mora and Galuscak 2022, p. 166; OECD Economic Outlook No 106 2019). In summary, people who were afraid of a new lethal virus had high expectations of the government, so the adoption of strict prevention measures even at the risk of economy was at least temporarily understandable.

With the goal of escaping from this health crisis as quickly as possible, the V4 leaders in power wanted the crisis to be de-politicized by their political foes or media, because the country had to be unified for the people ("us"). Thinking of the pandemic as a new opportunity to boost the legitimacy of populist governance, they further desired to brag about their crisis management skills and maintain popular support by demonstrating their dedication to the people ("us"). They instead stigmatized any critics and liberal media as traitors working for the political establishment and mainstream media at the national/EU level ("them"). On the basis of relatively high popular support, this populistic strategy ("us" vs. "them") appeared to work out in spring (Bene and Boda 2021; Cisar and Kubat 2021; Lipinski 2021; Sagan et al. 2022).

8.4 Narrative II: Why Did the V4 End Up Failing to Replicate the Success in the Fall?

Then how did the V4 fail in the fall? Just as the spring success was ascribed to a timely implementation of strict measures, the autumn failure was attributed to delayed and insufficient policy responses. Again, let us take a closer look at Figure 8.1. First of all, populist leaders missed the golden time in the fall. The SI before and after October was much lower than 50 in all Visegrad countries. In contrast, except for Austria, its level was at least around or above 50 in Western Europe. This contrast implies that the V4's pandemic policies were not that stringent in the second wave. Figure 8.1 demonstrates another interesting pattern. The policy stringency declined dramatically between April and October in the V4, while its drop in Western Europe during the same period was generally not as drastic. That is, Western Europe maintained a relatively higher level of stringency in the summer, whereas the V4 relaxed the severe measures shortly after the end of the first wave.

8.4.1 Escalation of Electoral Costs: Falling Public Confidence and Bad Economic Outlook

The lingering question is that if the three aforementioned factors (i.e., two institutional factors and popular support) contributed largely to the V4's relative success in the spring, then why did the V4 fail to respond swiftly and stringently in the fall? What changed? The main reason is that demand-side factors turned negative. In other words, the electoral costs of quick and stringent measures rose in the fall. Two institutional factors (i.e., strong executive capacity/autonomy and highly centralized epidemic-oriented healthcare system) remained the same in the fall, but public confidence was on the decline and the economic outlook became gloomy, so populist politicians in power did not respond properly to the second wave because of concerns over their falling popularity.

To begin with, public confidence in government and its preventive measures fell dramatically after late spring: Czechia: 62.5% → 40.7%; Hungary: 51.7% → 42.4%; Poland: 51.5% → 40.3%; Slovakia: 63.7% → 43% (European National Panels 2020). More than half the population supported each V4 government before the summer, but the level of public confidence dropped to around 40% approximately when the second wave arrived. The degree of panic also saw a rapid drop from 61.5%–77% in the first wave to 48.9%–64.7% in the second wave (European National Panels 2020). Thus, the V4 populist leaders had to pay attention to public mood swings. In this situation, it was very difficult for them to suddenly readopt health experts' scientific recommendations and reimpose strong restrictions on individual mobility, liberty, and socioeconomic activity. Populist policies are, as discussed earlier, characterized by an excessive sensitivity to the majority's opinions. The V4 leaders were therefore well aware that if they had reimplemented discredited strict measures, they would have been politically punished in the next election by the people.

Why did people become less concerned about the deadly impact of COVID-19 and not give strong support to their government's strict protective policies? Setting aside COVID-19 fatigue or tiredness, one main reason was the rising economic difficulties, such as job loss or insufficient state subsidies. People were no longer able to endure it. The OECD's economic outlook well describes the catastrophic state of the economy in 2020 (OECD Economic Outlook EO 107 2020) compared to 2019's positive GDP forecast (OECD Economic Outlook No 106, 2019). Public health was able to be prioritized at the expense of the economy in the spring, but the V4 leaders had to take economic hardship seriously in the fall. At this point, as mentioned earlier, health policies became subordinated to economic ones (Heinrich 2022, p. 44). However, to make matters worse, while self-praising their competent leadership, the V4 populists announced in the summer that the pandemic was over. In turn, people were already relaxed. In this situation, if the V4 leaders had suddenly reintroduced harsh policies that would have adversely affected the majority of people's daily lives, it was obvious that they would have had to take back their victory announcement and reconvince citizens to relive the tough times. As they were concerned about political backlash as a result of this rollback, they were unable to respond to the second wave swiftly.

8.4.2 *Ignored Science and Low Quality of Health Care*

On top of that, as electoral costs escalated, the V4's leaders did not or were unable to turn to expert advisory groups. They deactivated or curtailed the role of crisis management support teams working for the government after the first wave ended and reactivated those teams quite late after the beginning of the second wave (Sagan et al. 2022, p. 448; Steur 2021). In the meantime, as there was no more place for experts over the summer, science already lost its influence in politics (Sagan et al. 2022, p. 450). To be clear, it was not that significant even in the middle of the first wave, but at least leaders came up with guidelines based on scientific evidence (Bene and Boda 2021; Cisar and Kubat 2021; Lipinski 2021). As the epidemiological situation improved, however, they became less incentivized to depend on scientists' warnings. In turn, many ordinary citizens came to think that the pandemic would end soon. A mass dinner event held in Prague on June 30 exemplified this complacency, although the head of the WHO gave a strong warning message to the effect that "the worst is yet to come" beforehand. Thousands of people gathered to celebrate the end of the pandemic and shared food and drinks on the street (Meredith 2020). Neither leaders nor citizens listened to expert voices. In this regard, science was simply instrumental for the V4 populist leaders. Its value became much less important in politics once stringent NMIs became high-cost in electoral terms in the fall.

In the absence of the government-led stringent NMIs, the V4's healthcare systems were the only hope to hinder the spread of a strong infectious disease. However, it is well known that the overall quality of health care had been low for a long time. The V4 nonetheless reduced some measures over the summer (Sagan et al. 2022, pp. 451–453). After all, the issue of a shortage of qualified healthcare workers had not been resolved. As a result, as COVID-19 hit frontline doctors and nurses hard during the second wave, the V4 suffered severely from this problem in the fall. Several stopgap measures (e.g., volunteers, forcing medical students to work) were not sufficient to supplement professional medical staff (Sagan et al. 2022, 452; Sirotnikova et al. 2020). What is worse, the V4 did not even develop "effective find, test, trace, isolate, and support systems" (Sagan et al. 2022, p. 446), which might have been an efficient way to overcome the low quality of health care. To summarize, the V4's populist leaders in power were lax in predicting and preparing for the upcoming wave. The governments' short-term quick fixes overshadowed the aforementioned deep-seated healthcare deficiencies in the spring, but the issue of low-quality healthcare eventually came to the fore in the fall as governments failed to reimpose quick and strong restrictions, which led to a surge in the number of confirmed cases and deaths.

8.5 Conclusion and Discussion

Focusing on the political origins of the V4's COVID-19 policies in 2020, this essay finds that the spring success was attributable to a combination of two favorable institutional factors and high popular support and that the autumn failure was due to the fact that mass-level factors, despite the same institutional legacies, became hostile to the V4 populist leaders in government. In other words, the V4 retained a strong executive capacity/autonomy and highly centralized governance of the epidemic-oriented healthcare system in both the spring and fall; what changed in the second wave were inimical demand-side factors, namely, falling public confidence in government and its prevention measures and a dour economic outlook. As a consequence, as the escalation of electoral costs added to the political burden for incumbents, the V4's fall pandemic responses were neither timely nor sufficient to mitigate the spread of the virus. The Visegrad evidence reveals that populist leaders in power were equally responsive to their electoral incentives just like all election-minded politicians. They further enjoyed a greater capacity/autonomy for policy action when path-dependent post-Soviet legacies granted them organizational, administrative, and science-based procedural tools.

Overall, the V4's COVID-19 NMI policies relied heavily on executive leaders' decisions. Paradoxically, because of their successful experience in the spring, the V4 populist leaders in power became complacent over the summer. They no longer adhered to scientifically recommended policies and were thus ill-prepared for the second wave. Judging from this, it may be occasionally true that populist leaders with highly centralized governance can make a correct decision in times of crisis. Nevertheless, this kind of regime is still on shaky ground from a long-term crisis management perspective, because it hinges largely on the central leader's judgment calls and its policymaking mechanism is vulnerable to shifts in public opinion and other rapidly evolving circumstances (e.g., the fluctuations of electoral costs).

REFERENCES

Bayerlein M et al (2021) Populism and COVID-19: How populist governments (mis)handle the Pandemic. KIEL Working Paper No. 2192:1–44

Bene M, Boda Z (2021) Hungary: Crisis as usual – populist governance and the pandemic. In Bobba G, Hubé N (eds) Populism and the politicization of the COVID-19 crisis in Europe, Palgrave Macmillan, Switzerland Gewerbestrasse, p 87–100

Boot M (2020) Trump isn't the only populist leader losing the battle against the coronavirus. The Washington Post. https://www.washingtonpost.com/opinions/2020/05/06/trump-isnt-only-populist-leader-losing-battle-against-coronavirus. Accessed 1 Aug 2022

Bukowski P (2021) Poland's economy in the pandemic. The LSE Blog. https://blogs.lse.ac.uk/covid19/2021/10/18/polands-economy-in-the-pandemic. Accessed 1 Aug 2022

Buštíková L, Baboš P (2020) Best in Covid: Populists in the time of pandemic. Politics and Governance 8(4):496–508

Císaˇr O, Kubát M (2021) Czech Republic: Running the state like a family business. In Bobba G, Hubé N (eds) Populism and the politicization of the COVID-19 crisis in Europe, Palgrave Macmillan, Switzerland Gewerbestrasse, p 101–114

European National Panels (2020) National pandemic alarm https://www.nationalpandemicalarm.eu/en/2020-09-18?index=government_trust. Accessed 1 Aug 2022

Freedom House (2019) Freedom in the World 2019 Scores. https://freedomhouse.org/report/freedom-world/2019/scores. Accessed 1 Aug 2022

Gidengil E, Stolle D, Bergeron-Boutin O (2022) The partisan nature of support for democratic backsliding: A comparative perspective. European Journal of Political Research 61(4):901–929

Guasti P (2020) The impact of the COVID-19 pandemic in Central and Eastern Europe: The rise of autocracy and democratic resilience. Democratic Theory 7(2):47–60

Guasti P (2021) Democratic erosion and democratic resilience in Central and Europe during COVID-19. Czech Journal of International Relations 56(4):91–104

Heinrich A (2022) The Emergence of the Socialist Healthcare Model After the First World War. In Nullmeier F et al (eds) International Impacts on Social Policy: Global Dynamics of Social Policy. Palgrave Macmillan, p 35–46

Heller W et al (2023) The Institutional Underpinnings of Policy Making in the Face of the COVID-19 Pandemic in Europe In Shvetsova O [This volume]

Kavakli KC (2020) Did populist leaders respond to the COVID-19 pandemic more slowly? Evidence from a global sample. Working paper https://covidcrisislab.unibocconi.eu/sites/default/files/media/attach/Kerim-Can-Kavakli.pdf. Accessed 1 Aug 2022

Lindberg S (2018) The nature of democratic backsliding in Europe. Carnegie Europe https://carnegieeurope.eu/2018/07/24/nature-of-democratic-backsliding-in-europe-pub-76868. Accessed 1 Aug 2022

Lipin´ski A (2021) Poland: 'If we don't elect the president, the country will plunge into chaos'. In Bobba G, Hubé N (eds) Populism and the politicization of the COVID-19 crisis in Europe, Palgrave Macmillan, Switzerland Gewerbestrasse, p 115–129

Manaev G (2021) What did the USSR actually get right? Russia Beyond https://www.rbth.com/history/333668-what-did-ussr-actually-get-right. Accessed 1 Aug 2022

Mckee M et al (2021) Are populist leaders creating the conditions for the spread of COVID-19? International Journal of Health Policy and Management 10(8):511–515

Meredith S (2020) Thousands attend a street party in Prague to say goodbye to the coronavirus pandemic. CNBC https://www.cnbc.com/2020/07/01/coronavirus-thousands-attend-farewell-pandemic-party-in-prague.html. Accessed 1 Aug 2022

Meyer B (2020) Pandemic populism: An analysis of populist leaders' responses to COVID-19. Tony Blair Institute for Global Change https://institute.global/policy/pandemic-populism-analysis-populist-leaders-responses-covid-19. Accessed 1 Aug 2022

Milman O (2020) Trump administration cut pandemic early warning program in September. The Guardian https://www.theguardian.com/world/2020/apr/03/trump-scrapped-pandemic-early-warning-program-system-before-coronavirus. Accessed 1 Aug 2022

Mora M, Galuščák K (2022) Monetary and fiscal policy interactions in the wake of the pandemic: The case of the Czech Republic. BIS Papers 122:115–128

Mudde C (2004) The Populist Zeitgeist. Government and Opposition 39(4):541–563

Mudde C (2020) Will the coronavirus kill populism? Don't count on it. The Guardian https://www.theguardian.com/commentisfree/2020/mar/27/coronavirus-populism-trump-politics-response. Accessed 1 Aug 2022

Norris, P (2020) Global Party Survey, 2019. https://doi.org/10.7910/DVN/WMGTNS. Accessed 1 Aug 2022

OECD Economic Outlook EO 107 (2020) https://stats.oecd.org/Index.aspx?DataSetCode=EO107_EDITIONS. Accessed 1 Aug 2022

OECD Economic Outlook No 106 (2019) https://stats.oecd.org/Index.aspx?DataSetCode=EO106_INTERNET. Accessed 1 Aug 2022

PARLINE (2018) http://archive.ipu.org/parline-e/parlinesearch.asp. Accessed 1 Aug 2022

Phillips T (2020) Brazil's Jair Bolsonaro says coronavirus crisis is a media trick. The Guardian https://www.theguardian.com/world/2020/mar/23/brazils-jair-bolsonaro-says-coronavirus-crisis-is-a-media-trick. Accessed 1 Aug 2022

Rooduijn M et al (2019) The Populist: An overview of populist, far right, far left and Eurosceptic parties in Europe. https://popu-list.org. Accessed 1 Aug 2022

Sagan A et al (2022) A reversal of fortune: Comparison of health system response to COVID-19 in the Visegrad group during the early phases of the pandemic. Health Policy 126:446–455

Schecter K (1992) Soviet Socialized Medicine and the Right to Health Care in a Changing Soviet Union. Human Rights Quarterly 14 (2):206–215.

Sheiman et al (2018) The evolving Semashko model of primary health care: the case of the Russian Federation. Risk Management Healthcare Policy 11:209–220

Shvetsova O et al (2022) Protective Policy Index (PPI) global dataset of origins and stringency of COVID-19 mitigation policies. Scientific Data 9, 319. https://doi.org/10.1038/s41597-022-01437-9

Sirotnikova MG et al (2020) Central Europe: From pandemic exemplar to pariah. BalkanInsight https://balkaninsight.com/2020/10/15/central-europe-from-pandemic-exemplar-to-pariah. Accessed 1 Aug 2022

Steur M (2021) Slovakia's democracy and the COVID-19 pandemic: When executive communication fails. Verfassungsblog on Matters Constitutional https://verfassungsblog.de/slovakias-democracy-and-the-covid-19-pandemic-when-executive-communication-fails. Accessed 1 Aug 2022

Taggart PA (2004) Populism and Representative Politics in Contemporary Europe. Journal of Political Ideologies 9(3):269–288

The Oxford Coronavirus Government Response Tracker (OxCGRT) (2022) Covid-19: Stringency Index https://ourworldindata.org/covid-stringency-index. Accessed 1 Aug 2022

UNDP (2020) Human Development Report 2020 https://hdr.undp.org/system/files/documents/hdr2020pdf.pdf. Accessed Aug 2022

Urbinati N (2017) Populism and the Principle of Majority. In Kaltwasser CR et al (eds) The Oxford Handbook of Populism. Oxford University Press, p 571–589

V-Dem Institute (2019) V-Dem annual democracy report 2019. https://www.v-dem.net/documents/16/dr_2019_CoXPbb1.pdf. Accessed 1 Aug 2022

Visegrad Group (2022). https://www.visegradgroup.eu/about. Accessed 1 Aug 2022

Walters S (2020) Revealed: Boris Johnson scrapped Cabinet minister's pandemic team six months before coronavirus hit Britain. The Daily Mail https://www.dailymail.co.uk/news/article-8416075/Boris-Johnson-scrapped-Cabinet-Ministers-pandemic-team-six-months-coronavirus-hit-Britain.html. Accessed 1 Aug 2022

World Bank (2019a) GDP per capita (current US $). https://databank.worldbank.org/reports.aspx?source=2&series=NY.GDP.PCAP.CD&country=. Accessed 1 Aug 2022

World Bank (2019b) Employment in agriculture (% of total employment) (modeled ILO estimate) https://databank.worldbank.org/reports.aspx?source=2&series=SL.AGR.EMPL.ZS&country=. Accessed 1 Aug 2022

World Bank (2019c) Employment in industry (% of total employment) (modeled ILO estimate) https://databank.worldbank.org/reports.aspx?source=2&series=SL.IND.EMPL.ZS&country=. Accessed 1 Aug 2022

World Bank (2019d) Employment in services (% of total employment) (modeled ILO estimate) https://databank.worldbank.org/reports.aspx?source=2&series=SL.SRV.EMPL.ZS&country=. Accessed 1 Aug 2022

World Bank (2019e) Individual using the Internet (% of population). https://databank.worldbank.org/reports.aspx?source=2&series=IT.NET.USER.ZS&country=. Accessed 1 Aug 2022

World Health Organization (1998) Health Care Systems in Transition: Russian Federation https://www.euro.who.int/__data/assets/pdf_file/0014/120281/e72969.pdf. Accessed 1 Aug 2022

Zulianello M (2020) Varieties of populist parties and party systems in Europe: From state-of-the-art to the application of a novel classification scheme to 66 parties in 33 countries. Government and Opposition 55(2):327–347

CHAPTER 9

Common Law Systems and COVID-19 Policy Response: Protective Public Health Policy in the United States, Canada, New Zealand, and Australia

Michael Catalano and Aaron Chan

9.1 Introduction

COVID-19 presents challenges worldwide as the pandemic continues with more novel infections. Countries struggle with managing repeat infections, excess deaths, economic disruption, educational interruptions, and further political discord around policy responses. At the onset of the pandemic, policymakers experimented with policy responses with low levels of information about the COVID-19 virus and high levels of uncertainty about which public health measures and policies would best combat

---

M. Catalano (✉)
Department of Political Science, Binghamton University, Binghamton, NY, USA
e-mail: mcatala4@binghamton.edu

A. Chan
Binghamton University, Binghamton, NY, USA
e-mail: achan63@binghamton.edu

© The Author(s), under exclusive license to Springer Nature   197
Switzerland AG 2023
O. Shvetsova (ed.), *Government Responses to the COVID-19 Pandemic*, https://doi.org/10.1007/978-3-031-30844-4_9

the virus. Adding to the uncertainty, policymakers crafted policy with public opinion and the actions of other political institutions and policymakers in mind.

Policymakers in the executive and legislative branches, along with members of the bureaucracy, developed much of the policy response in the first year of the COVID-19 pandemic. However, these elements of government are not the only source of policy. The judiciary, particularly in common law legal systems, can amend, reject, and create policy. They tend to do so in a reactionary way—they act on legal cases and controversies based on the actions of other policymakers. Even so, the judiciary in countries play an important role in the policymaking process as a creator of policies and a veto player that may thwart the policies created by others.

To best understand the environment in which policymakers operated when responding to the COVID-19 pandemic, we pose the question: how do courts of last resort in common law legal systems function in the midst of a crisis? We would expect in "normal" times that different judicial ideologies would produce variation in how much courts of last resort constrain policy interventions that infringe on individual rights and movement, as was the case in COVID-19 mitigation efforts by government. Conservative policymakers, including judges, should want to constrain the powers of government; left-leaning policymakers should favor government intervention and policy to serve the public good. However, in times of crisis, policymakers, especially judges, must operate with low information and high uncertainty about implications of policy responses. In these instances, even conservative policymakers and courts may take a conciliatory stand on government intervention in crisis, allowing the government to use more powers than would be permitted in "normal" times.

In particular, we focus on the national courts of last resort in all four of the settler common law legal systems: the United States of America (US), Canada, New Zealand, and Australia. We explain that the ideology of the court matters in general in judicial decision-making; however, in environments with low information and high uncertainty amidst a crisis, judiciaries defer to other policymaking institutions responding to the crisis. When courts do act, they do so in response to policy that the court may not prefer. As a permission-granting institution, these courts can allow unpreferred policy to continue but limit its scope through the use of precedent.

As we detail further, we examine common law legal systems, rather than civil law legal systems, for three primary reasons. First, common law legal systems allow courts to create policy in a way that civil law legal system courts cannot. Second, the country cases here represent the entirety of British settler common law countries—it is a substantively exhaustive list.

Third, selected common law countries are paired with shared borders but different ideological leanings of national courts of last resort (i.e., USA-Canada and Australia-New Zealand).

Courts of last resort have final say on appeals; however, they have discretion in case selection and only hear and decide on a small percentage of cases. Lower courts create policy as well, especially in areas where courts of last resort have not decided. However, courts of last resort weigh disproportionately heavily in the considerations of other policymakers compared to their likelihood of exercising judicial review on policy. Given the supremacy of their answers to challenges, coupled with their outsized influence in the calculus of decision-making, it makes sense that we focus on courts of last resort.

In the context of the COVID-19 pandemic, national courts of last resort had an influence on how protective public health policy responses were considered in a court of law.[1] We define protective public health policies based on the work of Shvetsova et al. (2020a, 2021, 2022a, 2022b). Protective public health policies are defined as binding law and policy created in response to the COVID-19 pandemic in the following categories: states of emergency, border closures, school closures, social gathering and social distancing limitations, home-bound policies, medical isolation policies, closure/restriction of businesses and services, and mandatory personal protection equipment (PPE). These public health policies can come from a variety of sources, including legislation, executive action, or bureaucratic action and regulation.

With this foundation, when political actors of these respective countries make COVID-19 protective public health policies, the courts play a significant role in the policymaking process and calculus. Typically, challenges to COVID-19 response policies mean the courts have opportunities to rule on the legality of the policies. This means high courts have an ex post veto. Beyond that, with their ability to establish policy through binding precedent, high courts in common law systems can alter policy created by other actors to bring those policies closer to the ideal point of the courts.

This chapter addresses these issues by starting with an individualized examination of each of the four national courts of last resort of interest. Second, we provide important background information on each of

---

[1] Though courts exist among these countries at the national and subnational levels, the Supreme Court of the United States, Supreme Court of Canada, Supreme Court of New Zealand, and High Court of Australia will be the only courts discussed.

the four national courts of last resort, along with descriptions of these countries' political party systems. Third, we offer an explanation of the question we posed: how do courts of last resort in common law legal systems function in the midst of a crisis? Fourth, we explore the decisions of the national courts of last resort regarding COVID-19 policy responses. Finally, we offer a discussion and concluding thoughts.

9.2 National Courts of Last Resort in the United States, Canada, New Zealand, and Australia

The US, Canada, New Zealand, and Australia comprise the exhaustive list of former British settler colonies operating under a common law legal system. In these countries law is derived from judicial decisions instead of from statutes, as is the case in civil law legal systems. In other words, the law is defined by the legal rationale in the opinions and precedents created by courts through cases heard by those courts.

Each of these countries has multiple types of courts, distinguished by a variety of factors of jurisdiction including original versus appellate jurisdiction. Original jurisdiction courts, often referred to as trial courts, operate as fact-finding courts. They gather evidence and testimony and allow parties and their legal representation the forum to interact to determine winners in a case. Appellate courts, on the other hand, review cases previously decided by lower courts. These appellate courts do not attempt to uncover new facts on a case but monitor the process used by lower courts and the application of the law.

Courts of last resort reside as the final arbiters of disputes in the legal system. They establish binding precedent for all lower courts in their hierarchy. This makes courts of last resort incredibly influential in establishing and defining the law. However, the structure of these courts of last resort varies, as do the ways in which they operate, especially how they decide which cases to consider and rule on. We proceed with relevant descriptions of each of the four countries' courts of last resort and how they operate.

The Supreme Court of the US was established by the US Constitution and formed in 1789. The Court serves as the court of last resort on appeals, with limited original jurisdiction provided by the US Constitution. The US Supreme Court sits atop the federal judiciary, which contains general jurisdiction trial courts (US District Courts), intermediate appellate courts (US Court of Appeals), and numerous limited jurisdiction trial

9 COMMON LAW SYSTEMS AND COVID-19 POLICY RESPONSE: PROTECTIVE... 201

and appellate courts. Additionally, subnational state courts hold exclusive jurisdiction over all state matters that are not federal in nature. Supreme Court justices serve life tenure after selection by executive (presidential) appointment and confirmation by the upper chamber of the national legislature (US Senate).

The US Supreme Court has a discretionary docket and typically decides on only several cases each year. Cases where a majority of justices (usually out of nine) agree translate into precedent based on the opinion of the court. Most appeals come to the Supreme Court of the US through the process of writ of certiorari. In this process, a party asks the Supreme Court to request the record of their case for review from the lower court. In considering this application for writ of certiorari, the justices decide whether to hear and decide on the case or let the lower court ruling stand. Only four justices must vote to accept the case to place it on the docket.

The Supreme Court of Canada was established by an act of parliament in 1875 (the Supreme Court Act). The Canadian judiciary contains national- and subnational-level (provinces and territories) courts. The Supreme Court of Canada hears national-level appeals and appeals from territory/province-level courts of last resort. The court holds three sessions per year and hears between 65 and 80 appeals annually. Decisions in which a majority of the nine justices agree become binding precedent for all lower courts. After selection by the governor general of Canada (a representative of the British Commonwealth monarch) with advice from the Canadian prime minister, Canadian Supreme Court justices may serve until the mandatory retirement age of 75.

Most cases are appealed to the Supreme Court of Canada when a party applies to appeal the decision of a lower court. The party must obtain permission, or leave to appeal, from the court. In applications for leave of appeal, the Supreme Court of Canada makes a decision to grant or dismiss the appeal. If the court grants the appeal, then the appeal is heard with formal judgments setting the precedent coming either immediately after the decision is made (oral judgment) or at a time after (reserved judgment).[2]

The Supreme Court of New Zealand was established in 2004 by legislative statute. The court has appellate jurisdiction over areas prescribed by legislation enacted by the New Zealand Parliament. All appeals must come from the New Zealand Court of Appeals or High Court. Unlike the

---

[2] For more information on the appeals process in Canada, see: https://www.scc-csc.ca/case-dossier/stat/proc-eng.aspx.

202 M. CATALANO AND A. CHAN

federal structure of the US, Canada, and Australia, New Zealand operates as a unitary state, with no subnational units of government other than local governments. New Zealand's judicial hierarchy reflects this unitary structure, with all intermediate appellate courts, general jurisdiction trial courts, and limited jurisdiction courts being national level. Decisions become precedent when a majority of the justices (out of six) agree on an outcome and rationale. Justices serve life tenure after selection by the New Zealand attorney general, in consultation with the chief justice; the appointment process is managed by the Crown Law Office.

The Supreme Court of New Zealand decides very few cases each year, typically a dozen or less, due to the narrow area of jurisdiction set by the New Zealand legislature. The judicial review mechanism of the Supreme Court of New Zealand is substantially weaker than that of the other three countries in this chapter; the court can merely review the actions of the executive to determine whether she acted within the powers given to her by legislation. Appeals to the Supreme Court can be heard only with the leave of the court.[3] The court must not give leave to appeal unless it is satisfied that it is necessary in the interests of justice for the court to hear and determine the proposed appeal.[4]

Finally, the High Court of Australia was established by the Constitution of Australia in 1901. The High Court of Australia possesses both original and appellate jurisdiction over all elements of Australian law. The Australian judiciary contains intermediate appellate courts and trial courts at the national and subnational (state) levels. These subnational state and territory courts have jurisdiction over matters of state law and, in some instances, federal law. As with the other countries discussed in this chapter, decisions become binding precedent when a majority of justices considering a case agree with the outcome and rationale. After appointment by the governor-general in council (a representative of the British Commonwealth

---

[3] For more information on the appeals process in New Zealand, see: https://www.courtsofnz.govt.nz/the-courts/supreme-court/how-cases-are-heard/.

[4] It is necessary in the interests of justice for the Supreme Court to hear and determine a proposed appeal if:

- the appeal involves a matter of general public importance;
- a substantial miscarriage of justice may have occurred, or may occur, unless the appeal is heard;
- the appeal involves a matter of general commercial significance; or
- the appeal involves a significant issue relating to the Treaty of Waitangi.

9 COMMON LAW SYSTEMS AND COVID-19 POLICY RESPONSE: PROTECTIVE... 203

monarch), justices on the High Court of Australia may remain in their role until the mandatory retirement age of 70.

Appeals to the High Court of Australia can come from lower national (federal) courts and the courts of last resort for states and territories. Typically, each year has several dozen cases decided from appeal or special leave application, with less than a dozen on the original jurisdiction docket. There is no automatic right to have an appeal heard by the High Court, and parties who wish to appeal must persuade the court in a preliminary hearing that there are special reasons to cause the appeal to be heard. Decisions of the High Court on appeals are final. There are no further appeals once a matter has been decided by the High Court, and the decision is binding on all other courts throughout Australia.[5]

9.3 POLITICAL PARTIES AND COURTS OF LAST RESORT IN THE SETTLER BRITISH COMMONWEALTH COUNTRIES

Judiciaries do not operate in a vacuum; they consider the actions of other members of the political environment (Epstein and Knight 1998). This includes political parties; political parties work to control the policymaking components of the state, including the judiciary, in an attempt to established preferred policy as law. Political parties hold various levels of influence over the judiciary, specifically through selection and retention methods (Bonica and Sen 2021a). These levels of political party influence over parties create various ex ante and ex post controls over courts, which can alter outcomes in legislation (Catalano 2022) and judicial decision-making. We proceed with a brief overview of the political party systems in each country, which establishes the basis for our measure of ideology of justices for this chapter.

The four Settler British Commonwealth countries generally boast two-party (or coalition) systems, with power alternating between center-left and center-right parties (Table 9.1). In the US, the party system is dominated by the center-left Democratic Party and center-right to rightist Republican Party. Broad coalitions of interest groups comprise both parties. Furthermore, these parties have exhibited evidence of polarization, particularly at the elite level. Political parties attempt to "capture" the

---

[5] For more information on the appeals process in Australia, see: https://www.hcourt.gov.au/about/operation-of-the-high-court#:~:text=Each%20Justice%20makes%20his%2Fher,Court%20at%20a%20later%20sitting.

204　M. CATALANO AND A. CHAN

Table 9.1 Political party systems and ideology in Settler British Commonwealth countries

Ideology	United States	Canada	New Zealand	Australia
Leftist		New Democratic and Green	Green	
Center-left	Democratic	Liberal	Labour	Labor
Centrist		Bloc Québécois (independence)	Maori (Indigenous rights)	
Center-right	Republican	Conservative	National	Liberal and nationals
Rightist			ACT	

judiciary through selection mechanisms by controlling the executive branch (presidency) and legislative chambers (Senate) (Bonica and Sen 2021a).

There are five major national parties in Canada, with power shifting largely between the Liberal Party (center-left) and Conservative Party (center-right). Three smaller parties are also represented in the Canadian Parliament: the New Democratic Party (NDP) (leftist), Bloc Québécois (independence), and Green Party of Canada (leftist). Though the national parties have state-level party organizations, these parties may have some separation in the hierarchical organization. In general, there is limited evidence of polarization between the parties, especially when compared to the US.

The New Zealand legislature also hosts members of five political parties. As in Canada, party often shifts between the center-left party (Labour) and the center-right party (National), with smaller parties like the Green (leftist), ACT (rightist), and Maori (centrist, indigenous rights) comprising the remainder of the seats of the New Zealand Parliament. Given the unitary structure of the New Zealand government, the political parties in New Zealand take on a largely centralized structure as well. New Zealand political parties display relatively limited polarization (Satherley et al. 2020).

In Australia, a "mild" two-party system exists, with the Liberal Party (center-right) and Nationals (center-right) forming a coalition opposing the center-left Labor Party. While the balance of power often rests between

9 COMMON LAW SYSTEMS AND COVID-19 POLICY RESPONSE: PROTECTIVE... 205

these two parties/coalitions, more than ten percent of members of parliament come from minor parties or are unaffiliated with a political party. As in the US and Canada, there exists a connection between national- and state-level party organizations. Commentators on Australian politics have said that polarization is growing slightly but is somewhat mitigated by a ranked-choice voting system in national parliamentary elections (Singer 2022).

9.4 MAPPING PARTISANSHIP AND IDEOLOGY ON COURTS OF LAST RESORT

Ideology matters when considering judicial decision-making and the outcomes of cases. The question is often not whether ideology matters, but rather how much it factors into judicial decision-making compared to extra-judicial factors. For some scholars, justices on national courts of last resort with high levels of judicial independence may decide according to their sincere preference, making judicial ideology paramount in understanding judicial behavior (Segal and Spaeth 2002). Others argue that justices must act strategically, considering the actions and preferences of others (e.g., legislatures, executives, the public) when making decisions and not relying solely on their individual ideology (Epstein and Knight 1998). In this chapter, we argue that, while ideology matters, justices must act strategically in the context of the greater policymaking environment. Specifically, justices must consider how their preferences map onto situations and cases when information is low and uncertainty of implications is high, as was the case in the early part of the COVID-19 pandemic.

The courts of last resort vary in terms of the partisanship and ideology of the justices. Tables 9.2, 9.3, 9.4, and 9.5 represent the sitting justices of the highest court of the US, Canada, New Zealand, and Australia in 2020, respectively. While more sophisticated measures of judicial ideology exist,[6] none span the set of countries we consider in this chapter. As a result, we opt for a more comprehensive measure of ideology using the partisanship of the appointing government of each individual justice on the court of last resort as an indicator of that individual justice's ideology. A number of studies have taken this approach, specifically in the US context (Gottschall 1983; Tomasi and Velona 1987). Indeed, Pinello (1999) finds that

---

[6] See, for example, from studies of the US judiciary: Bonica and Sen (2017, 2021b), Epstein et al. (2007), Johnston et al. (2016), Windett et al. (2015).

206 M. CATALANO AND A. CHAN

Table 9.2 Ideological identification of Supreme Court of United States in 2020

Justice's name	Nominator's name	Political affiliation of nominator	Political affiliation of justice
John G. Roberts, Jr	George W. Bush	Republican Party	Republican Party
Clarence Thomas	George H. W. Bush	Republican Party	Republican Party
Ruth Bader Ginsburg[a]	Bill Clinton	Democratic Party	Democratic Party
Stephen G. Breyer	Bill Clinton	Democratic Party	Democratic Party
Samuel A. Alito, Jr	George W. Bush	Republican Party	Republican Party
Sonia Sotomayor	Barack Obama	Democratic Party	Democratic Party
Elena Kagan	Barack Obama	Democratic Party	Democratic Party
Neil M. Gorsuch	Donald Trump	Republican Party	Republican Party
Brett M. Kavanaugh	Donald Trump	Republican Party	Republican Party
Amy Coney Barrett+	Donald Trump	Republican Party	Republican Party

Note: This table represents the members of the US Supreme Court in 2020, their nominators, and each person's political affiliation

[a]Ruth Bader Ginsburg served on the Supreme Court of the US until her death on September 18, 2020. She had been active in deliberations and decisions up until her death. + Amy Coney Barrett succeeded Ruth Bader Ginsburg on October 27, 2020, and began hearing and deciding on cases at that time

Table 9.3 Ideological identification of Supreme Court of Canada in 2020

Justice's name	Nominator's name	Political affiliation of nominator	Political affiliation of justice
Rosalie S. Abella	Paul Martin	Liberal Party	Liberal Party
Richard Wagner	Justin Trudeau	Liberal Party	Liberal Party
Michael J. Moldaver	Stephen Harper	Conservative Party	Conservative Party
Andromache Karakatsanis	Stephen Harper	Conservative Party	Conservative Party
Suzanne Côté	Stephen Harper	Conservative Party	Conservative Party
Russell Brown	Stephen Harper	Conservative Party	Conservative Party
Malcolm Rowe	Justin Trudeau	Liberal Party	Liberal Party
Sheilah L. Martin	Justin Trudeau	Liberal Party	Liberal Party
Nicholas Kasirer	Justin Trudeau	Liberal Party	Liberal Party

Note: This table represents the members of the Canadian Supreme Court in 2020, their nominator, and each person's political affiliation

9 COMMON LAW SYSTEMS AND COVID-19 POLICY RESPONSE: PROTECTIVE... 207

Table 9.4 Ideological identification of Supreme Court of New Zealand in 2020

Justice's name	Nominator's name	Political affiliation of nominator	Political affiliation of justice
Helen Winkelmann	David Parker	Labour Party	Labour Party
Susan Glazebrook	Chris Finlayson	National Party	National Party
Mark O'Regan	Chris Finlayson	National Party	National Party
Ellen France	Chris Finlayson	National Party	National Party
Joe Williams	David Parker	Labour Party	Labour Party
William Young	Chris Finlayson	National Party	National Party

Note: This table represents the members of the New Zealand Supreme Court in 2020, their nominators, and each person's political affiliation

Democratic (the center-left party in the US) judges decide cases in a left-leaning direction, while Republican (the center-right party in the US) judges decide cases in a right-leaning direction.

As established earlier in this chapter (see the section "National Courts of Last Resort in the United States, Canada, New Zealand, and Australia), each of these national courts of last resort has justices nominated by the executive branch of the government (though confirmation processes do vary). As with the judiciary, we use the ideological positions of the parties' relevant policymakers as proxies for their ideology. Therefore, in determining the ideology of individual justices, we use the party of the nominating executive branch at the time of appointment as the indicator for that individual justice. Furthermore, when discussing the parties in cases around COVID-19 policies later in this chapter, we will use the same party system structure to determine the divergence of ideology between justices on a court of last resort and the policymaker of the policy in dispute in the particular case.

In the following set of tables (Tables 9.2, 9.3, 9.4, and 9.5), each table displays the members of the respective court, their nominating/appointing entity, the nominator's political affiliation, and the justices' political affiliation. This demonstrates the composition of each court and helps define ideology to better understand whether a court is considered more liberal, conservative, or perhaps neutral where party affiliation is equally divided among the court.

A majority of justices sitting on the Supreme Court of the US in 2020 were nominated by Republican presidents (Table 9.2). The court grew

Table 9.5 Ideology identification of the High Court of Australia in 2020

Justice's name	Nominator's name	Political affiliation of nominator	Political affiliation of justice
Michelle Gordon	Tony Abbott	Liberal Party	Liberal Party
Stephen Gageler	Julia Gillard	Labor Party	Labor Party
Patrick Keane	Julia Gillard	Labor Party	Labor Party
Simon Steward[a]	Scott Morrison	Liberal Party	Liberal Party
Susan Kiefel	John Howard/Malcolm Turnbull	Liberal Party	Liberal Party
James Edelman	Malcolm Turnbull	Liberal Party	Liberal Party
Geoffrey Nettle[a]	Tony Abbott	Liberal Party	Liberal Party

Note: This table represents the members of the Australian High Court in 2020, their nominators, and each person's political affiliation

[a]Justice Steward succeeded Justice Nettle in November 2020

more conservative across 2020 after Justice Ruth Bader Ginsburg (appointed by a Democratic president) passed away in office and was replaced by Justice Amy Coney Barrett (appointed by a Republican president) in the latter part of 2020. The conservative majority has been skeptical of government intervention across a variety of fronts in the policymaking environment in the US.

The Supreme Court of Canada had a majority of justices (five) appointed by the Liberal Party, indicating a left-leaning majority on the court (Table 9.3). In general, Liberals tend to be more permissive of government interventions compared to Conservatives, though neither party exhibits the same level of polarization as in the US. Members of the Liberal Party treated COVID-19 policy responses more favorably compared to members of the Conservative Party, though there was bipartisan support for the COVID-19 policy response in the early months of the pandemic in Canada (Merkley et al. 2020; Pickup et al. 2020). We would expect this to hold for justices on the Supreme Court of Canada.

While New Zealand operated a common law system before 2004, the selection methods for its court of last resort changed in 2004. As such, defining the ideology of the court of last resort in New Zealand presents challenges that do not exist in the other three countries examined in this chapter. Since 2004, the New Zealand attorney general has consulted with the chief justice before making appointments to the New Zealand Supreme Court. The attorney general is a member of the executive branch, reporting to the prime minister of New Zealand. As such, the attorney general is a member of the prime minister's party and can be considered an agent of the prime minister. Based on party affiliations of the appointing attorney general, we see New Zealand has a solid center-right majority of National Party-appointed justices (Table 9.4).

Finally, the High Court of Australia was held by a majority (4 to 2) of Liberal Party-appointed members through 2020. This established a solid center-right majority on the High Court. Table 9.5 displays seven justices because Justice Steward succeeded Justice Nettle in November 2020. Both of these justices were nominated by the Liberal Party Prime Minister, meaning the partisan composition of the court did not change.

9.5 Courts of Last Resort During Crisis: Low Information and High Uncertainty

In our explanation, we answer our question posed at the onset of this chapter: how do courts of last resort in common law legal systems function in the midst of crisis? After presenting our base assumptions, we argue that justices have preferences (ideology) they work to install as policy through precedent born out of case outcomes. However, justices must act strategically and consider extra-judicial factors when deciding cases, like the conditions of the COVID-19 pandemic. We proceed with our argument that times of crisis mean policymakers operate in an environment with low information and high uncertainty. Courts have incentive to act cautiously in checking government action and policy interventions, even when such action and interventions infringe on individual rights and movement, as was the case in protective policy responses to the COVID-19 pandemic. However, courts can still act to grant or deny permission to policymakers or narrow the scope of the policy if the court does not prefer said policy but remains uncertain on implications of altering the status quo. We conclude this section with our theoretical expectations.

First, we establish our base assumptions for our theory. This theory specifically considers courts of last resort in common law systems. We assume that courts are policymaking institutions (Dahl 1957). We assume that common law appellate courts (including courts of last resort) react to other policymaker actions. These courts cannot proactively thwart policy; rather, these courts must wait for challenges to policy to work their way through the legal system until appealed to the court. This offers first-move advantages to other policymakers. Next, we assume that it is costly for courts to act and decide on challenged policy. Courts must expend time and resources when hearing and deciding cases; furthermore, action carries the risk of reaction by other policymakers or perceptions of unfairness by the public. Lastly, we assume that judges act strategically in attempts to secure preferred policy outcomes (Epstein and Knight 1998). While we assume that judges are policy-seeking actors, we argue that to achieve policy goals, they must also consider the preferences of other policymakers, the social impact of their decisions, and public perceptions of legitimacy.

Ultimately, judges care about policy outcomes. When presented with the opportunity, judges prefer to establish policy closer to their ideal point. In general, left-leaning policymakers (such as judges) favor government interaction on behalf of the public good. Meanwhile, right-leaning policymakers prefer to limit government intervention in order to preserve individual rights. Courts tend to act on these broad preferences within external constraints based on the ideological composition of judges on the court.

Judges act strategically as they attempt to secure preferred policy outcomes. Strategic decision-making means judges consider other policymakers' preferences, the social impact of their decisions on the public, and public perceptions of legitimacy of the court. In the policy realm, courts can consider two general scenarios of ideological congruence with or divergence from other policymakers. In a unified government scenario, where courts and other policymakers are ideologically congruent, the court can act on challenges to strengthen the policy as precedent or choose not to act. In either case, the status quo (preferred policy) remains. The choice to act, however, creates costs on the court, while not acting still renders the preferred outcome with no cost to the court. Meanwhile, in a divided government scenario, where courts and other policymakers are ideologically divergent, the court may act to overturn the policy or narrow the scope of the policy in its impact. Not acting means an unpreferred status quo remains in place.

Judges must also act strategically based on perceptions of the public, even when the court is not directly accountable to the public. In particular, judges understand that case outcomes can carry implications for society and perceived legitimacy of the court. Court decisions can have real impacts on society. Decisions may alleviate stresses from society, exacerbate issues in society, or otherwise alter the way society operates. Judges tend not to want to have broad, rapid, transformative impacts on society based on individual decisions.

Connected to social impact, judges recognize the need to maintain public perceptions of legitimacy. Legitimacy acts as an enforcement mechanism for judicial decisions; a public that perceives the judiciary as legitimate acts as a credible threat to policymakers who shirk judicial decisions (Vanberg 2005). To shirk judicial decisions means policymakers do not follow the case law set by those court decisions.

Judges must also consider external factors beyond other policymakers or the public when making decisions. Times of crisis and emergency create a unique set of circumstances jolting courts out of their typical decision-making process. We define crisis as "a state of affairs in which a decisive change for better or worse is imminent… [in] times of difficulty, insecurity, and suspense in politics or commerce."[7] Decisive action implies that time horizons for action in crisis may be short; shortened time horizons alter the incentives and behaviors of policymakers compared to "normal" times with longer time horizons (Olson 1993). As the COVID-19 virus spread exponentially throughout the world, policymakers operated under short time horizons, understanding each day mattered in attempting to mitigate and prevent this spread.

Difficulty in a situation can stem from a lack of information on the situation and its implications. During the early months of the COVID-19 pandemic, information on the virus and its consequences proved sparse. For most of 2020, medical professionals, public health experts, and policymakers alike had little knowledge of the virus, how it spread, and what mitigation efforts they could use to prevent the virus. A lack of information inspires uncertainty over the future and implications of actions taken to mitigate the crisis. Higher levels of uncertainty create the "insecurity and suspense" in crisis.

In times of emergency and crisis, society demands a response from policymakers to deliver society from the crisis it faces. Policymakers must answer the demands from society and respond to the crisis with protective policy aiming to protect members of society from the consequences of the

---

[7] We derive our definition from the Oxford English Dictionary (https://www.oed.com/view/Entry/44539?redirectedFrom=crisis#eid). Last accessed: December 19, 2022.

212 M. CATALANO AND A. CHAN

crisis while attempting to resolve the issues presented by the crisis. Policymaking in crisis is often made by executives, who can invoke emergency powers and work quickly to address the emergency expediently. They are often followed by legislatures, who may alter or grant legitimacy to existing policy and create new policy responses.

Judiciaries also make policy in crisis. They must continue to operate in general to resolve disputes, some of which challenge policies aiming to resolve the crisis at hand (Matyas et al. 2022). Unlike executives and legislatures, judiciaries tend not to be directly accountable to the public; therefore, they can defer to other policymaking entities and not act in crisis, when information is low and uncertainty is high.

Indeed, judiciaries have incentives to not act in crisis. First, they are not as well equipped as other policymaking entities to respond to crisis. Second, nonaction means courts will not incur costs from the public for making mistakes in the crisis. Third, judiciaries understand that the crisis will eventually pass, as will the heightened need for government intervention.

With these incentives in mind, courts considering challenges to policy created by ideologically divergent policymakers may wait to overturn less preferred policy after the emergency has passed. Alternatively, if these courts do act during the emergency, they may do so to grant permission for the policy but ensure that this policy is narrow in its implementation so that it does not become precedent for future emergencies or during "normal" times. In other words, with divided government (courts v. executive/legislature) the court needs to give permission for policy to continue. With a unified government (courts aligned with executive/legislature), the court does not need to incur the costs to offer permission as it already prefers the status quo.

This brings us to our expectations. With high uncertainty and low information, we expect courts to act cautiously (or not act at all) while the crisis is ongoing. Each country discussed in this chapter (US, Canada, New Zealand, and Australia) set protective policy at the national and sub-national levels in response to the COVID-19 pandemic in 2020 (Adeel et al. 2020; Shvetsova et al. 2022c). We expect that left-leaning national courts of last resort will not act on challenges to COVID-19 protective policies in 2020, regardless of whether the source of the policy was from a left-leaning or right-leaning policymaker. Alternatively, we expect that right-learning courts will tend not to act on challenges to COVID-19 protective policies. However, if a right-leaning court does act, it would do

9 COMMON LAW SYSTEMS AND COVID-19 POLICY RESPONSE: PROTECTIVE... 213

so with respect to policy set by ideologically divergent policymakers. In those instances, we expect that right-learning courts will tend to grant permission to left-leaning policymakers but do so in a way to narrow the scope, duration, or legacy of the challenged policy.

9.6 ANALYSIS OF DECISION-MAKING BY NATIONAL COURTS OF LAST RESORT IN CRISIS

Two of our four national courts of last resort decided cases on the merits involving COVID-19 protective polices in 2020 (Table 9.6).[8] The US Supreme Court and Australian High Court, the two most conservative (right-leaning) courts of last resort in this analysis, decided five cases on the merits, upholding government action of subnational policymakers four times out of the five. In each instance, the subnational government was led by left-leaning parties that were ideologically divergent from the national court of last resort. We analyze each case in this section and continue the discussion in the "Discussion" section of this chapter.

9.6.1 United States of America

In the US, as in other common law countries, courts give themselves the discretion to review existing policy and create new policy. The US Supreme

---

[8] It is important to note that each of our four countries of interest saw some challenges to COVID-19 protective policy responses land in their national judiciary, even if they did not rise to the national court of last resort in 2020. In the United States, a number of cases were decided by the Supreme Court through its use of the emergency docket (also known as the "shadow docket"). The Supreme Court rarely used the emergency docket until very recently. Decisions in this process do not receive oral arguments and are not arrived at on the merits, with little precedential value for lower courts and future cases (Badas et al. 2022). In Canada, interest groups, like the Canadian Civil Liberties Association, monitored cases of violations of individual rights through protective policy responses from the onset of the pandemic, with an eye to challenging these violations in the Canadian judiciary (Deshman 2020). In New Zealand, the Court of Appeals (intermediate appellate court) considered two cases involving the national lockdown (*Borrowdale v. Director-General of Health [2020] NZCA 156 8 May 2020* and *Nottingham v. Ardern [2020] NZCA 144 4 May 2020*). The High Court of New Zealand (national general jurisdiction trial court) decided a number of cases as well on COVID-19 protective policies in 2020 (see https://www.courtsofnz.govt.nz/judgments/covid-19-related-judgments/). In Australia, the High Court of Australia showed discretion in its selection of cases related to COVID-19 protective polices in 2020, as in the United States.

214   M. CATALANO AND A. CHAN

Table 9.6 Counts of COVID-19 policy response cases decided on the merits in 2020

Country	No. of COVID policy cases	No. of cases that upheld COVID-19 policy response
United States	3	2
Canada	0	0
New Zealand	0	0
Australia	2	2

Court had established the precedent of responding to pandemic policy in the landmark case *Jacobson v. Massachusetts* (1905). In this case, the court decided that the state had the power to compel vaccinations to protect the public health and safety of citizens.[9] The US Supreme Court added to this line of case law regarding pandemic policy through the three COVID-19 policy-related cases it decided in 2020: *South Bay United Pentecostal Church v. Newsom* (2020), *Calvary Chapel Dayton Valley v. Sisolak* (2020), and *Roman Catholic Diocese of Brooklyn v. Cuomo*.

In *South Bay United Pentecostal Church v. Newsom* (2020), the right-leaning Supreme Court declined to block a California executive order, established by a left-leaning policymaker, which placed temporary numerical restrictions on public gatherings. It also blocked part of the executive order where it restricted any gathering that surpassed 25 percent capacity or up to 100 people in places of worship. This protective policy attempted to limit gathering sizes, especially those held indoors and consistent with meetings such as churches. The disagreement in this case was that the First Amendment right of religious free exercise was infringed upon. Yet, in a five-to-four vote, the court upheld the California policy.

Less than two months later, in July 2020, the Supreme Court delivered the majority opinion on *Calvary Chapel Dayton Valley v. Sisolak* (2020). The court again declined to block a Nevada executive order, set by a left-leaning policymaker, that limited attendance at religious services. The order refused more than fifty persons to any one religious service despite the fact that other venues, including casinos, were permitted to have up to fifty percent capacity. This case was brought as a challenge to the policy that it violated the US Constitution's First Amendment's religious free

---

[9] *Jacobson v. Massachusetts* (1905): https://www.oyez.org/cases/1900-1940/197us11.

exercise clause. Like the previously discussed case, the vote was 5–4 with the dissenting Justices being Thomas, Alito, Gorsuch, and Kavanaugh.

Near the end of 2020, the Supreme Court of the US departed from precedent and overturned policy set by a left-leaning policymaker in *Roman Catholic Diocese of Brooklyn v. Cuomo* (141 S. Ct. 63 [2020]). Between this case and *Calvary Chapel Dayton Valley v. Sisolak*, left-leaning Justice Ruth Bader Ginsburg passed away and was succeeded by right-leaning Justice Amy Coney Barrett. The Roman Catholic Diocese of Brooklyn challenged a restriction on large gatherings for places of worship in New York as an infringement on the First Amendment. The policy was established by left-leaning policymaker Andrew Cuomo. Unlike in the prior two cases, the court overturned the protective policy (Parmet 2021).

9.6.2 Canada

In Canada, the Supreme Court acts as the court of last resort, where it has jurisdiction over arguments in constitutional, administrative, criminal, and civil law. The Canadian Supreme Court does not hold trials but instead listens to appeals from other appeals courts. In 2020, the Supreme Court of Canada did not receive any cases disputing any COVID-19 public policy responses in any province or at the national level. There were some provincial cases, but they never advanced to the court.

This does not necessarily mean that the court did not care to listen to any cases regarding COVID-19 responses, it just means that none had reached the court. Other appellate courts did settle disputes. However, no challenge to policy found its way to the Supreme Court docket in 2020 testing its constitutionality. And while there are no cases to analyze and reflect on opinions, we can still theorize how cases may have gone in the first several months of the pandemic in Canada's court of last resort.

Unlike the conservative bench of the Supreme Court of the US, the majority of Canada's court is liberal leaning. A more left-leaning court would likely result in more restrictive COVID-19 protective public health responses being upheld in court. However, given the support for pandemic policy response across the political spectrum in Canada, the political elites may have determined that challenging policy, at least early on in the pandemic, would not provide political benefits for their party. With challenges less likely due to widespread public and elite support, this enabled policymakers to craft responses and tackle COVID relatively free of political pushback from the judiciary or public.

9.6.3 New Zealand

Similar to Canada, New Zealand had no COVID-19 policy challenge that reached its national court of last resort. The Supreme Court of New Zealand only hears cases the judges grant leave to appeal, and none that matched the six types of responses focused on this chapter reached the court in 2020. Furthermore, New Zealand's Supreme Court has a narrower jurisdiction over cases, set by the national legislature. This means that many COVID-19 protective policy disputes settled in lower appeals courts may not have been under the Supreme Court's jurisdiction.

As New Zealand has become more progressively liberal over the years, the court has remained more conservative. The fact that cases were settled at lower appeals courts doesn't really allow us to determine patterns or actions by this bench composition. Labour Party-aligning justices would prioritize public health and well-being, while National Party-aligning justices would push for individual freedoms and less restrictive public health policies. However, as also seems to be the case here, lower courts upheld policies and the Supreme Court was not asked to further question anything. This enabled New Zealand to mitigate COVID-19 within communities throughout the country without any political obstacles. It is fair to say that this judicial support made handling COVID-19 primarily science based, and that lines up with records on how New Zealand handled the first COVID wave.

9.6.4 Australia

The right-leaning High Court of Australia considered two cases involving COVID-19 protective policy in 2020. In both instances, the court upheld government interventions by left-leaning policymakers at the subnational level. This appears to support our theoretical expectations. When the first wave of the pandemic hit Australia, both the states and federal government jumped in, implementing protective public health policies to best mitigate the outbreak. This inherently limits individual liberties by telling citizens to quarantine, imposing a curfew, telling people to wear face masks, and deciding whether they can even travel or not. This issue of movement appears at the heart of both *Palmer v. Western Australia* (2020) and *Gerner v. Victoria* (2020).

In November 2020, the court heard *Palmer v. Western Australia*. In May of that year, Clive Palmer was not allowed to enter Western Australia

9 COMMON LAW SYSTEMS AND COVID-19 POLICY RESPONSE: PROTECTIVE... 217

due to an order closing the subnational border to all nonessential travelers. Mr. Palmer challenged this policy, citing section 92 of the Australian Constitution, which he argued guaranteed that "trade, commerce, and intercourse among the States" shall be "absolutely free." The policy was put in place by the Labor-led (left-leaning) state government of Western Australia. The right-leaning High Court of Australia determined that the policy did not violate the constitution in emergencies "constituted by the occurrence of a hazard in the nature of a plague or epidemic," narrowing the scope of future government action in this area.

A month later, in December 2020, the court reviewed *Gerner v. Victoria* (*Gerner v. State of Victoria* [2020] HCA 48). In this case, a small business owner (Gerner) challenged the constitutionality of the lockdown policy established by the left-leaning Labor Party-led subnational government in Victoria. As in *Palmer v. Western Australia*, Gerner invoked section 92 of the Australian constitution, arguing that the restriction on movement impacted his business. Again, the right-leaning High Court of Australia upheld the COVID protective policy established by the left-leaning policymakers in Victoria. These results demonstrate that Australia's policymakers, even those ideologically divergent from the right-leaning High Court of Australia, received permission to continue protective policies against the pandemic.

9.7 Discussion and Conclusion

Protective policy responses to COVID-19 brought conflict between and among national- and state-level policymakers. The federal nature of governments created informational and authority redundancies that allowed multiple levels of policymakers to issue responses to the COVID-19 pandemic (Shvetsova et al. 2020b). The variation in who decides how to respond to health crises created differences in health outcomes and public opinion (Shvetsova et al. 2022a, 2022b; VanDusky-Allen et al. 2022).

The protective policy responses set public health interventions in conflict with individual rights. Policies related to travel restrictions, stay-at-home orders, the wearing of PPE, and following social distancing rules were mandatory, and limitations on social gatherings, school closures, and restrictions on restaurants, nonessential businesses, and other venues all tested the limits of executive and legislative powers in dealing with an unprecedented health crisis. These policies created the potential for a multitude of cases for courts to consider. While cases did arise, the national courts of last resort did not act very often to decide these cases on the merits.

In the four British settler common law judiciaries (US, Canada, New Zealand, and Australia), only five cases were considered in 2020, the first year of the COVID-19 pandemic. In four of these five cases, right-leaning national courts of last resort upheld policy responses by left-leaning sub-national policymakers. In upholding these policies, the right-leaning courts tended to write opinions that narrowed the long-term implications of the policies once the pandemic passed.

These courts of last resort followed a general pattern of not disturbing executive decision-making during the earliest part of the COVID-19 pandemic. At this time in the emergency, courts like other policymakers operated in an environment of low information and high uncertainty. Courts had an incentive to not incur costs of decision-making in these conditions, whereas other policymakers did not have such a luxury.

Though common law courts of last resort tended not to act or meddle in executive action regarding COVID-19 policies, we did see differences emerge along ideological lines. Right-leaning courts needed to say whether they opposed government action and had to give permission for interventions they would have likely not supported in "normal" times. Left-leaning courts did not have to give permission because they preferred government intervention no further action was required on their part. In other words, with government divided between courts and other policymakers, courts need to give permission. And in a unified government (where courts align with executives and legislators), courts do not need to incur costs to grant permission.

This chapter addresses the overarching need to understand judicial decision-making in times of crisis. Our argument and subsequent analysis support the nascent literature on this topic born largely out of the COVID-19 pandemic. The stance of judicial nonintervention in Australia and Canada followed the precautionary principle, where serious risk of harm and uncertainty should not preclude government responses (Webber 2022). When courts must make decisions during emergencies, with low information, they tend to defer to other policymakers and minimize the impact the court might have (Silverstein and Hanley 2009–2010). However, when determining whether or not to take up cases on the docket, judges must decide whether emergencies justify more restrictions than would otherwise be permitted under "normal" circumstances and

9 COMMON LAW SYSTEMS AND COVID-19 POLICY RESPONSE: PROTECTIVE... 219

which rights deserve more protection compared to others (Madera 2022; Mariner 2021).

Many variables that were not tested could be further examined to continue this line of research. The personal characteristics of judges has been shown to alter judicial decision-making in times of crisis (e.g., Collins et al. 2008). External factors, outside the exogenous crisis, also need to be considered beyond judicial ideology. With the impact that decisions regarding responses to crises can have on society, courts consider how society might be impacted and how society might perceive the court's actions. Concern over social implications and consequences for the legitimacy of the court may explain why right-leaning US Chief Justice John Roberts voted with the left-leaning justices on the US Supreme Court. It has been noted how Chief Justice Roberts has concerned himself with nurturing the legitimacy of the US judiciary. Knowing the potential negative consequences of overturning temporary government interventions in an emergency, Chief Justice Roberts opted to uphold policies and preserve trust in the court rather than risk deepening the crisis by overturning said policies.

While no one hopes for a crisis or emergency, especially like the COVID-19 pandemic, we must still prepare for such eventualities. Public health policies are not set by executives, legislatures, and bureaucrats in a vacuum; they must consider the constitutionality of said policies, especially when there are implications for individual rights and government powers. It is imperative to understand the mechanics behind judicial decision-making in times of crisis so that policymakers can administer effective AND legal policies to mitigate and prevent emergencies.

References

Adeel, Abdul Basit, Michael Catalano, Olivia Catalano, Grant Gibson, Ezgi Muftuoglu, Tara Riggs, Mehmet Halit Sezgin, Olga Shvetsova, Naveed Tahir, Julie VanDusky-Allen, Tianyi Zhao, and Andrei Zhirnov. 2020. "COVID-19 Policy Response and the Rise of the Sub-National Governments." *Canadian Public Policy* 46(4): 565–84.

Badas, Alex, Billy Justus, and Siyi Li. 2022. "Assessing the Influence of Supreme Court's Shadow Docket in the Judicial Hierarchy." *Justice System Journal.* https://doi.org/10.1080/0098261X.2022.2143304.

Bonica, Adam, and Maya Sen. 2017. "A Common-Space Scaling of the American Judiciary and Legal Profession." *Political Analysis* 25(1): 114–121.

Bonica, Adam, and Maya Sen. 2021a. The Judicial Tug of War: How Lawyers, Politicians, and Ideological Incentives Shape the American Judiciary. Cambridge, UK: Cambridge University Press.

Bonica, Adam, and Maya Sen. 2021b. "Estimating Judicial Ideology." *Journal of Economic Perspectives* 35(1): 97–118.

Catalano, Michael. 2022. "Ex Ante and Ex Post Control over Courts in the US States: Court Curbing and Political Party Influence." *Justice System Journal.* https://doi.org/10.1080/0098261X.2022.2123287.

Collins, Paul, Daniel Norton, Kenneth Manning, and Robert Carp. 2008. "International Conflicts and Decision Making on the Federal District Courts." Justice System Journal 29(2): 121–144.

Dahl, Robert. 1957. "Decision-making in democracy: The supreme court as national policy-maker." *Journal of Public Law* 6(2): 279–295.

Deshman, Abby. 2020. "A Civil Liberties Take on Canada's Second Wave of COVID-19 Emergency Orders." *Canadian Civil Liberties Association/ Association Canadienne des Libertes Civiles.* November 19. Last Accessed: December 21, 2022.

Epstein, Lee, and Jack Knight. 1998. *The Choices Justices Make.* Washington, DC: CQ Press.

Epstein, Lee, Andrew Martin, Jeffrey Segal, and Chad Westerland. 2007. "The Judicial Common Space." *Journal of Law, Economics, and Organizations* 23(2): 303–325.

Gottschall, J. 1983. "Carter's Judicial Appointments: The Influence of Affirmative Action and Merit Selection on Voting on the U.S. Court of Appeals." *Judicature* 67: 164.

Johnston, Christopher, Maxwell Mak, and Andrew Sidman. 2016. "On the Measurement of Judicial Ideology." *Justice System Journal* 37(2): 169–188.

Madera, Adelaide. 2022. "Governments' Legal Responses and Judicial Reactions during a Global Pandemic: Preliminary Remarks." Journal of Church and State 64(4): 551–561.

Matyas, David, Peter Wills, and Barry Dewitt. 2022. "Imagining Resilient Courts: from COVID-19 to the Future of Canada's Court System." Canadian Public Policy/Analyse de politiques 48(1): 186–208.

Merkley, E., Bridgman, A., Loewen, P., Owen, T., Ruths, D., & Zhilin, O. (2020). A Rare Moment of Cross-Partisan Consensus: Elite and Public Response to the COVID-19 Pandemic in Canada. Canadian Journal of Political Science, 53(2), 311–318. https://doi.org/10.1017/S0008423920000311.

Mariner, Wendy. 2021. "Shifting Standards of Judicial Review During the Coronavirus Pandemic in the United States." German Law Journal 22(6): 1039–1059.

Olson, Mancur. 1993. "Dictatorship, Democracy, and Development." *American Political Science Review* 87(3): 567–576.

9 COMMON LAW SYSTEMS AND COVID-19 POLICY RESPONSE: PROTECTIVE... 221

Parmet, Wendy. 2021. "Roman Catholic Diocese of Brooklyn v. Cuomo – The Supreme Court and Pandemic Controls." New England Journal of Medicine 384(3): 199–202.

Pickup, M., Stecula, D., & Van der Linden, C. (2020). Novel Coronavirus, Old Partisanship: COVID-19 Attitudes and Behaviours in the United States and Canada. *Canadian Journal of Political Science*, 53(2), 357–364. https://doi.org/10.1017/S0008423920000463.

Pinello, Daniel. 1999. "Linking Party to Judicial Ideology in American Courts: A Meta-analysis." *Justice System Journal* 20(3): 219–254.

Satherley, Nicole, Lara Greaves, Danny Osborne, and Chris Sibley. 2020. "State of the nation: trends in New Zealand voters' polarisation from 2009–2018." *Political Science* 72(1): 1–23.

Shvetsova, Olga, Andrey Zhirnov, Abdul Basit Adeel, Mert Can Bayar, Onsel Gurel Bayrali, Michael Catalano, Olivia Catalano, Hyoungrohk Chu, Frank Giannelli, Ezgi Muftuoglu, Dina Rosenberg, Didem Seyis, Bradley Skopyk, Julie VanDusky-Allen, and Tianyi Zhao. 2022c. "Protective Policy Index (PPI) global dataset of origins and stringency of COVID 19 mitigation policies." *Sci Data* 9, 319. https://doi.org/10.1038/s41597-022-01437-9.

Shvetsova, Olga, Julie VanDusky-Allen, Andrei Zhirnov, Abdul Basit Adeel, Michael Catalano, Olivia Catalano, Frank Giannelli, Ezgi Muftuoglu, Dina Rosenberg, Mehmet Halit Sezgin, and Tianyi Zhao. 2021. "Federal Institutions and Strategic Policy Responses to COVID-19 Pandemic." *Frontiers in Political Science* 3:631363. https://doi.org/10.3389/fpos.2021.631363.

Shvetsova, Olga, Andrey Zhirnov, Abdul Basit Adeel, Michael Catalano, Olivia Catalano, Hyoungrohk Chu, Garrett K Dumond, Georgian-Marius Ghincea, Jason Means, Ezgi Muftuoglu, Tara Riggs, Almira Sadykova, Mehmet Halit Sezgin, Julie Vandusky Allen, and Tianyi Zhao. 2020a. "Constitutional and Institutional Structural Determinants of Policy Responsiveness to Protect Citizens from Existential Threats: COVID-19 and Beyond.

Shvetsova, Olga, Andrei Zhirnov, Julie VanDusky-Allen, Abdul Basit Adeel, Michael Catalano, Olivia Catalano, Frank Giannelli, Ezgi Muftuoglu, Tara Riggs, Mehmet Halit Sezgin, Naveed Tahir and Tianyi Zhao. 2020b. "Institutional Origins of Protective COVID-19 Public Health Policy Responses: Informational and Authority Redundancies and Policy Stringency", Journal of Political Institutions and Political Economy: Vol. 1: No. 4, pp 585–613. https://doi.org/10.1561/113.00000023.

Shvetsova, Olga, Andrei Zhirnov, Frank Giannelli, Michael Catalano, and Olivia Catalano. 2022a. "Governor's Party, Policies, and COVID-19 Outcomes: Further Evidence of an Effect." *American Journal of Preventive Medicine* 62(3): 433–37.

Shvetsova, Olga, Andrei Zhirnov, Frank Giannelli, Michael Catalano, and Olivia Catalano. 2022b. "Can Correlation Between Governor's Party and COVID-19

Morbidity Be Explained by the Differences in COVID-19 Mitigation Policies in the States?" *American Journal of Preventive Medicine* 62(6): e381–e383.

Silverstein, Gordon, and John Hanley. 2009–2010. "The Supreme Court and Public Opinion in Times of War and Crisis." Hastings Law Journal 61(6): 1453–1502.

Singer, Peter. 2022. "How Australia Revived the Political Middle." *Project Syndicate* June 7. https://www.project-syndicate.org/commentary/australia-ranked-choice-voting-mitigates-polarization-by-peter-singer-2022-06. Last Accessed: December 15, 2022.

Segal, Jeffrey, and Harold Spaeth. 2002. *The Supreme Court and the Attitudinal Model Revisited.* New York, NY: Cambridge University Press.

Tomasi, T. B., and J. A. Velona. 1987. "All the President's Men? A Study of Ronald Reagan's Appointments to the U.S. Court of Appeals." *Columbia Law Review* 87: 766.

Vanberg, Georg. 2005. *The Politics of Constitutional Review in Germany.* Cambridge, UK: Cambridge University Press.

VanDusky-Allen, Julie, Steven Utych, and Michael Catalano. 2022. "Partisanship, Policy, and Americans' Evaluations of State-Level COVID-19 Policies Prior to the 2020 Election." *Political Research Quarterly* 75(2): 479–496. https://doi.org/10.1177/10659129211056374.

Webber, Katie. 2022. "The precautionary principle and judicial decision making in the COVID-19 pandemic." Australian Journal of Administrative Law 29(1): 43–59.

Windett, Jason, Jeffrey Harden, and Matthew E. K. Hall. 2015. "Estimating Dynamic Ideal Points for State Supreme Courts." *Political Analysis* 23(3): 461–469.

CHAPTER 10

Commonalities and Differences in Governments' COVID-19 Public Health Responses Around the World

Olga Shvetsova and Andrei Zhirnov

10.1 Introduction

The year 2020 tasked politicians with navigating a pandemic the likes of which had not been experienced for a century. Their response was not uniform: there was significant variation both in the politics and processes of pandemic decision-making and the resulting stringency and content of nonmedical interventions (NMIs). In the preceding chapters of this volume, the authors analyzed and compared the approaches chosen by political incumbents around the world, offered possible explanations of the differences, and delivered empirically grounded theoretical insights.

O. Shvetsova (✉)
Department of Political Science and Economics, Binghamton University, Binghamton, NY, USA
e-mail: shvetso@binghamton.edu

A. Zhirnov
University of Exeter, Exeter, UK
e-mail: A.Zhirnov@exeter.ac.uk

© The Author(s), under exclusive license to Springer Nature Switzerland AG 2023
O. Shvetsova (ed.), *Government Responses to the COVID-19 Pandemic*, https://doi.org/10.1007/978-3-031-30844-4_10

223

In this chapter, we take stock of the key points already made in the volume. Building on these insights, we also make broader comparisons and provide a general picture of the patterns of politicians' behaviors during the pandemic. Perhaps more fittingly with the arguments of the contributors, here we also take note of the aspects of the pandemic response where patterns were absent and differences dominated in the global policy landscape.

Political economy looks for fundamental theoretical explanations of strategic behaviors, such as the behaviors of politicians when in office, mindful that the incentives and constraints are set for the actors by the rules of the game in which they won their incumbency. A clear takeaway that emerged in all chapters is that the decision-making around NMIs in 2020 was at least in part driven by the political motives and not just considerations of public health: political incumbents pursued their political agendas as they chose and implemented the public health measures. The resulting biases in the strength of the policy interventions, our contributors suggest, could go both ways. Political expediency made some incumbents reluctant to implement unpopular and/or politically risky public health policy restrictions. But it inspired others to crank up the stringency of their pandemic policies and use them, e.g., to suppress the political challenges they faced.

Constitutions and the institutions governing the making of public policies in general and public health regulations in particular somewhat constrained who could and could not act in response to the pandemic, what kinds of decisions they were eligible to make, and what steps they needed to take to adopt given policies. In electoral democracies, politicians' choices were also constrained by the fear of electoral backlash against unpopular policies. Finally, politicians had to face economic realities and limitations of their countries' healthcare infrastructure.

The remainder of this essay is organized as follows. Rather than revisiting each of the preceding chapters one by one, we discuss their findings in four blocks: (1) constraints imposed by constitutions and political institutions, (2) the characteristics of governing parties and party systems, (3) economic constraints, (4) constraints imposed by the limited access to healthcare.

10.2 Political Institutions and Pandemic Decision-Making

10.2.1 Decentralization and Federalism

Political decentralization and federalism were brought into high relief by many accounts of pandemic management, and among them are four of the chapters in this volume (VanDusky-Allen 2023; Adeel and Zhirnov 2023; Bayrali 2023; Zhao 2023). The general fascination with federalism during the pandemic happened for two reasons. First, as an institutional parameter, federalism and decentralization did, overall, positively correlate with the stringency and adaptability of pandemic public NMIs. Figure 10.1 uses Protective Policy Index (PPI) data (Shvetsova et al. 2022; see the data description in Chap. 1 and Appendix A, Tables A1 and A2) to illustrate the point. In it, countries' daily overall PPIs (vertical axis) are plotted for the period between February and September 2020 (horizontal axis). We see in Fig. 10.1 that federations (solid line) produced a stronger policy response in February–March than nonfederations (dotted line) and maintained it at a higher level on average later in that prevaccine year, even though the NMIs' stringency fluctuated according to epidemiological need. Note that Fig. 10.1 excludes the countries that were nonfree as of 2019 (Freedom House 2020).

The second reason the political accounts of pandemic management pay so much attention to federalism and decentralization is that, in much of the world, governments at different levels played what looks like a tug of war when it came to adopting the NMI policies and, consequently, to shouldering the blame for the hardships created during the crisis. While only one set of NMIs, be it via national, state/provincial, or county-level policies, is required to protect the public, among the national, subnational, and local governments the question arose as to who would produce these necessary policies and thus bear the political responsibility for them. VanDusky-Allen (2023, Chapter 3) shows that, where policy production was not centralized, where the national executive had refrained from adopting stringent NMIs, cooperation and coordination among the different levels of government could proceed with varying levels of effectiveness, and the coordination failures could lead to efficiency losses. Her essay exposes the broader issue with policy coproduction in federations and decentralized polities: even though the abundance of decision makers who could, in principle, impose protective policies in a given domain could lead to (harmless) policy duplication and ensure a necessary

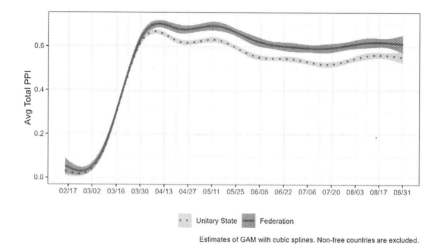

Fig. 10.1 Daily (Average Total) Protective Policy Index in Federal versus Unitary Countries, February–August 2020. (Source: Shvetsova et al. (2022), Freedom House (2020); author coding of federations.)

minimum level of policy provision, it may also result in inefficiently low policy output.

Figures 10.2 and 10.3 demonstrate this using a large N sample. Figure 10.2 shows average national PPI (horizontal axis) plotted against average regional PPI (vertical axis) on four different dates during 2020. Country observations that are above the positive diagonal have subnational-level governments that are more active than the national government. Below the diagonal, the national level is more active than the subnational level.

Figure 10.3 displays the contributions of subnational and national governments to the total of the NMI stringency and policy overlap/duplication between them in the production of NMIs. It plots the average national PPI as a share of total PPI (or how much, relatively speaking, the national level was doing on its own, horizontal axis) against average regional PPI as a share of total PPI (or how much, relatively speaking, the subnational governments were doing by themselves, vertical axis), for the same four dates in 2020 as in Fig. 10.2.

Note that this allows us to compare the relative contributions of the levels of government in NMI policy production, regardless of how

10 COMMONALITIES AND DIFFERENCES IN GOVERNMENTS' COVID-19... 227

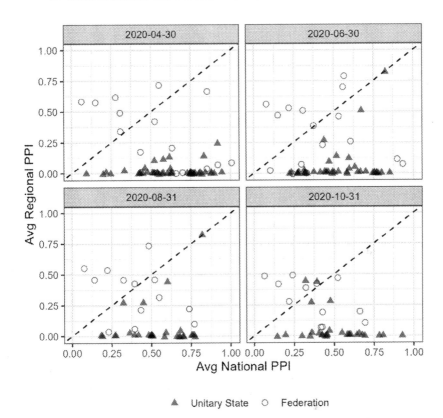

Fig. 10.2 NMI policy efforts of national and subnational governments on four dates in 2020. (Source: Shvetsova et al. (2022), Freedom House (2020); author coding of federations.)

stringent the overall protections were. If governments divided responsibilities exactly, observations should be on the dashed line, on the negative diagonal. Almost all federations are, however, above the negative diagonal, reflecting the fact that both levels of government introduced NMIs, and in the same policy categories. We observe policy duplication in NMI production, but we do not consider this to be inefficient; instead, we consider this productive duplication. Political duplication served as a useful system redundancy and protected against policy failure; it was a guarantee

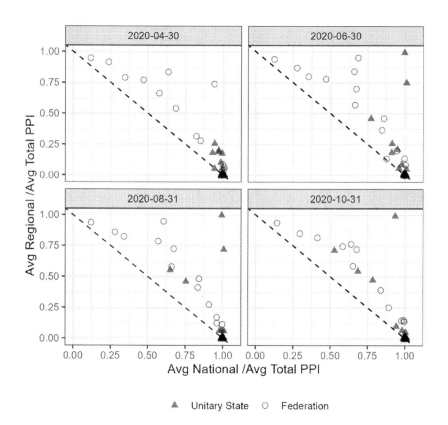

Fig. 10.3 Relative policy contribution to overall NMI stringency by national and subnational governments on four dates in 2020. (Source: Shvetsova et al. (2022), Freedom House (2020); author coding of federations.)

that a NMI would be in place for the population even if the other levels of government had failed to act.

One might think that coordination among the levels of government would depend on how well the respective jurisdictions and the coordination procedures were spelled out in the countries' legal and constitutional framework. Adeel and Zhirnov (2023, Chapter 4) demonstrate that clear division of roles is not sufficient to ensure intergovernmental coordination. Even though on paper India and Pakistan had similar divisions of responsibilities in the event of a public health emergency, in India the coproduction of policies by the state and federal governments was smoothed by the existing practices of intergovernmental collaboration in the areas of economic planning and development. In Pakistan, such practices were not developed, and provincial and federal governments ended up at odds over pandemic-related decision-making.

In Bayrali's (2023, Chapter 5) account of cooperation across the levels of government of South Africa and Nigeria, the integrating role was played by political parties. Policy coproduction displayed different patterns in party systems with and without strong national-subnational electoral and career linkages. The presence of strong national-subnational linkages among the party elites in South Africa compelled the national executive to step in and absorb the political costs of producing the NMI policies. In contrast, in Nigeria, in the absence of such party linkages, the national government, to a large extent, refrained from taking any action, pushing much of the burden of responsibility onto the subnational and local incumbents. This idea also resonates with one of the conclusions drawn by VanDusky-Allen (2023, Chapter 3): in Latin American federations, different party affiliations of the incumbents were one of the factors explaining the poor coordination across the levels of government.

Chapter 6 by Zhao (2023) further explores the variation in the policy response among decentralized polities and focuses on the pandemic politics in Indonesia and Malaysia. He departs from prior findings that pandemic management was more decentralized in federations compared to unitary countries and demonstrates that the general pattern was reversed if we compare Malaysia and Indonesia. Even though Malaysia is a federation and Indonesia is a unitary state, contrary to expectations, the policy response was much more centralized in Malaysia. Zhao's argument links the strategies of Joko Widodo in Indonesia and Muhyiddin Yassin in Malaysia not with the political institutions that assign and constrain their respective governments' responsibilities, but with the political pressures of the moment and the presence of binding economic constraints. The boundaries surrounding executive action or inaction in an emergency that institutions and constitutions might draw can be so wide that they hardly act as binding constraints on politicians' choices. In such cases, the momentary considerations of incumbents and their political opportunism can become the true drivers of their crisis mitigation strategies.

As these contributions show, there were significant differences among federations in how much governments at different levels cooperated in the production of NMIs and contributed to the overall stringency of the policy response. The large N cross-national comparison in Fig. 10.4 lends further credence to this result, demonstrating a substantial variation within, rather than across, the federal and unitary subsamples.

10.2.2 Separation of Power

All authors report that the bulk of pandemic NMI policies was produced by the executive branch, at all levels of government. The power of executives lies in their direct links to the machinery that implements policies, produces public services, and is involved in the day-to-day business of government. Another factor is that, unlike the legislation passed by parliaments, executive policy production was relatively simple. Parliaments are complex—possibly bicameral, possibly with specialized committees, and possibly constrained by the executive and judicial vetoes. Formal processes for executive decisions are uncomplicated in comparison. Most of the constitutions vest the executive branch with responsibilities to act in emergencies, and at the same time they empower the legislatures and the judiciary with passive emergency powers—the powers to review and reverse executive actions and set boundaries. Appendix B, Fig. B.1 compares this predominantly executive in origin policy production in parliamentary versus presidential democracies.

Catalano and Chan (2023, Chapter 9) scrutinize the role of the judiciary in pandemic-related policymaking in four common law countries, the United States, Canada, Australia, and New Zealand, and find little evidence of the judiciary intervening with executive decision-making. Despite the differences in political leanings, justices either refused to adjudicate or upheld the decisions of the executives. Adeel and Zhirnov (2023, Chapter 4) give an example of an unusual involvement of Pakistan's Supreme Court in pandemic decision-making that reinforces this point: the judiciary had to intervene only because of the failure of intergovernmental coordination.

10.2.3 Democracies and Autocracies

The authors here do not raise the issue of the difference in NMI policies between full and partial democracies in their comparative samples. Large N analysis conforms with this: as shown in Fig. 10.5, the speed and stringency in the adoption of public health policies were similar in partial and full democracies and superior to those in nondemocracies. Another interesting and potentially theory-extending observation is that both

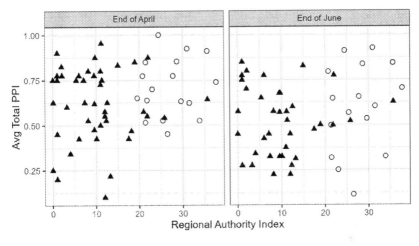

Fig. 10.4 Protective policy stringency (average total PPI) and decentralization and federalism, April and June 2020. (Source: Shvetsova et al. (2022), Freedom House (2020), Shair-Rosenfield et al. (2020), Hooghe et al. (2016); author coding of federations.)

democracy and decentralization were associated with more frequent changes in the protective policy stringency in 2020. These political system types thus demonstrated a higher sensitivity of policy measures to the changing environments—informational, epidemiological, and political.

10.3 Political Parties and Party Systems

10.3.1 Party Systems

As the discussion in the preceding section suggests, constitutions and institutions are not the only constraints on emergency policymaking. In electoral democracies, political incumbents face political pressure from their parties and their voters, and those do not necessarily push them in the same direction. As Bayrali (2023) in Chapter 5 argues, the reelection needs of copartisans at another level of government can push politicians to

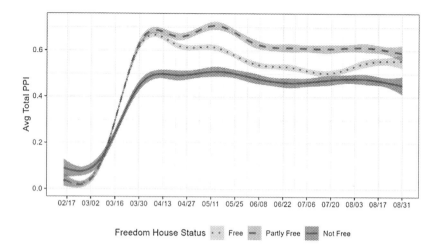

Fig. 10.5 Daily (average total) PPI in free, partly free, and nonfree countries, February–August 2020. (Source: Shvetsova et al. (2022), Freedom House (2020).)

take action in situations where they would otherwise avoid taking political risks.

Heller et al. (2023) in Chapter 2 argue that multiparty governments produce policies of higher stringency when their member parties are not in direct competition with each other. Contrary to the conventional wisdom, they found that power sharing in coalition cabinets improved the speed and stringency of crisis response. Their explanation lies in the stronger "political capital" held by smaller parties with strong roots in their constituencies that, as a rule, comprise multiparty governments, which enabled those governments to adopt painful policies at lower political cost to themselves.

The dynamics that Heller et al. (2023) identify in their small n most-similar comparison is not apparent in a broader sample where the choice of control variables is limited (Appendix B, Figs. B2 and B3), though not refuted. The strong and convincing findings from the theoretically focused case study analysis in Heller et al. (2023) highlight the value of the methodology of the small n most-similar-case perspective, which allowed the authors to avoid overspecifying their model.

10.3.2   Did Populism Impede Pandemic Response?

Two of the chapters, by Bayar and Seyis (2023, Chapter 7) and Cho (2023, Chapter 8), raise the question of whether the governments led by populist politicians systematically differed in their response to the pandemic. Populists are known to offer political solutions that on the surface address the most pressing issues as felt by the majority of voters but may be less concerned about causing detrimental long-term effects. Arguably, they were reluctant to implement policies that could protect public health if it meant curtailing any economic activity (Naushirvanov et al. 2022). The authors demonstrate that populist executives were extremely sensitive to the preferences of the population and tailored their NMI strategies to what their publics would be most likely to accept. This observation reinforces Heller et al.'s (2023, Chapter 2) theoretical argument that difficult choices and leadership in the crisis were best displayed where parties in power had a long-term, strong connection to their core constituencies. In combination, these findings suggest an agenda for future research: do institutionalized parties and party systems (Mainwaring and Scully 1995) have an increased capacity to address societal crises, as those inevitably come up, and thus improve political regimes' resilience and societies' welfare?

That said, the actual NMI policies that populists put in place during the pandemic varied considerably. Our contributors demonstrate that the policies formulated by populist incumbents depended on the particulars of the type of populist at the helm of a given country's executive branch, as well as institutional constraints and popular perceptions. Some of the variation could be attributed to coordination successes or failures in policy coproduction between the federal and subnational governments (VanDusky-Allen 2023, Chapter 3). There was also a difference in administrative epidemic preparedness, which increased the policy capacity for East European populist executives (Chu 2023, Chapter 8). In addition, and most importantly, popular attitudes varied, and where the public expected a proscience response, the proscience response was produced (Bayar and Seyis 2023, Chapter 7), yet only for as long as the population remained broadly on board (Chu 2023, Chapter 8).

10.4 Economic Constraints

Our contributors also discuss two types of noninstitutional but still politically relevant constraints that affected the willingness of governments to introduce more stringent NMIs. Stringent NMIs inevitably reduced the volume of economic activity in the national economies, slashing incomes and jeopardizing the ability of daily wage earners to earn a living. All contributors in this volume stress the tradeoffs that political incumbents faced between accountability for adverse health outcomes and more immediate backlash for economic hardships imposed.

Zhao (2023, Chapter 6) points out that the level of economic development beyond just gross domestic product (GDP) played a role in constraining governments, whereby the use of some NMIs was not feasible because of employment and education patterns. VanDusky-Allen (2023, Chapter 3) and Zhao (2023, Chapter 6) attribute at least part of the greater stringency in the policies made in Argentina and Malaysia (in comparison to other countries in their regions) to their relatively strong economies.

Using a broader sample, Fig. 10.6 illustrates the relationship between the income category of a nation, as defined using the standard World Bank classification, and the average policy stringency over the period of the first six months of the pandemic. Economic constraints in low-income countries may have proven binding, as evident in the global sample as well, and limited the feasible stringency of adopted NMIs.

10.5 Access to Healthcare and the Substitution Effect Between NMIs and Healthcare

Notably, although the practice of healthcare financing and provision clearly mattered, it was not identified by any of the authors in this volume as a crucial determinant of politicians' strategies. Politics rather than public health practice drove politicians' decisions to enact NMIs. Still, Fig. 10.6 reveals an interesting pattern. While the initial response was similar (note that "not free" countries are excluded in Fig. 10.7), when information improved, the NMI stringency fell in countries with public healthcare financing (following both the single-payer national health service and social health insurace models of health financing) but remained very high in countries where voluntary insurance is the prevalent model of healthcare financing. Was this because the population was more vulnerable

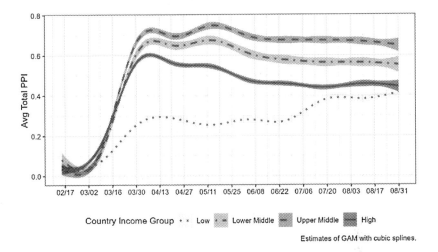

Fig. 10.6 Daily (average total) PPI by country income group, February–August 2020. (Source: Shvetsova et al. (2022); the country income group is computed using gross national income (GNI) per capita, PPP (The World Bank, World Development Indicators 2020).)

and had less access to treatment if sick in private health insurance systems? This phenomenon, under-theorized at present, requires an explanation in future research.

One explanation of this result is that the public's access to curative health care could reduce the pressure to impose nonmedical restrictions. As was discussed in Chap. 1, we theorize that politicians do not like to be responsible for policies that impose public health restrictions—hardship and mandates—on their constituents. They will only go as far in NMI stringency as is necessary to avoid excessively negative health outcomes for the public or the collapse of the healthcare system's capacity, both of which are not only normatively undesirable but also potentially politically dangerous for incumbents.

Consistent with that theory, there appears to have been a substitution effect, where reduced healthcare capacity was being made up for by more stringent NMIs. This may have happened for two reasons: a country's healthcare system can provide simultaneous care to a larger share of the population in countries where the capacity is greater, and the public in countries with greater healthcare capacity is more confident in the quality

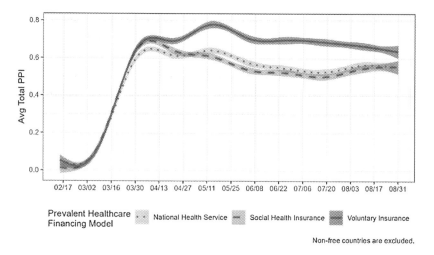

Fig. 10.7 Daily (average total) PPI in countries with different healthcare financing models, February–August 2020. (Sources: Shvetsova et al. (2022), Freedom House (2020); author coding of healthcare models.)

of care that they would receive if infected and so they show lower demand for the prevention of infections through NMIs. This substitution effect, theoretically, should have become even stronger when vaccine distribution began and the global inequalities in vaccine access came to the fore. We leave the enquiry into the causal mechanisms for this phenomenon to future researchers and here report the observation of such a substitution effect.

Figure 10.8 shows general trends in NMI stringency (vertical axes) by absolute per-capita government spending on health care in 2019 for the end of April and June of 2020. While on the whole a negative trend (substitution effect) is evident on both dates, it is more pronounced in June, when there was a clearer understanding of the scope of the public health threat that COVID-19 posed, versus in April, when, absent such information, precautionary behavior (Gollier 2001) as reflected in NMI adoption dominated.

Figure 10.8 demonstrates the same phenomenon but using the indicator of per-capita numbers of doctors and nurses in 2019 (horizontal axes) as a proxy for the capacity of a healthcare system, since the government spending indicator might not capture in full the variation in total

10 COMMONALITIES AND DIFFERENCES IN GOVERNMENTS' COVID-19... 237

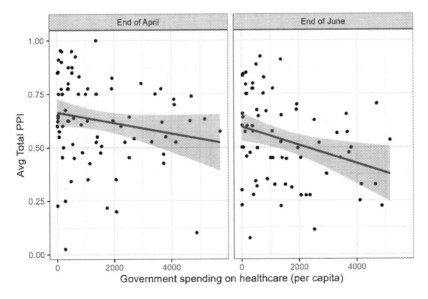

Fig. 10.8 Government per-capita healthcare spending in 2019 and the protective policy stringency (average total) in April and June 2020. (Sources: Shvetsova et al. (2022), World Health Organization (2020a).)

healthcare expenditures. The patterns from Fig. 10.9 are essentially replicated with this alternative measure: higher healthcare capacity resulted in weaker preventive policies, especially outside of the initial low-information phase.

The significance of the right to health care or some other form of constitutional guarantees of health care cannot be overstated in any discussion of access and utilization of health care. Even more intriguing is the apparent lack of a correspondence between the presence of such guarantees in a country's constitution and the stringency of the NMIs that were adopted during the prevaccine pandemic period (Fig. 10.10). Should not the constitutional guarantees create stronger accountability for political incumbents when it comes to the health of the population? This, again, is a puzzle for future researchers to solve.

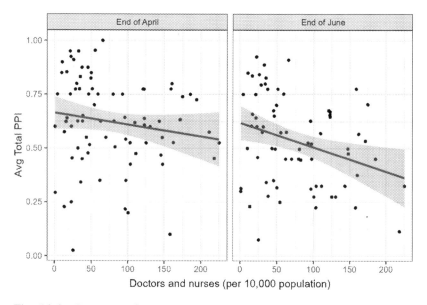

Fig. 10.9 Doctors and nurses per 10,000 people in 2019 and the protective policy stringency (average total) in April and June 2020. (Sources: Shvetsova et al. (2022), World Health Organization (2020b).)

10.6 Conclusion

Arguably, the world is entering an era of increased frequency of global health crises and natural disasters under an ever-present threat of climate change. How we govern ourselves matters for the ways in which we will live through these difficult times. Better policy production might mean better outcomes for all of us (Appendix B, Fig. B4). The authors in this volume make some observations backed by mixed-method analysis on the many ways in which government organization and political realities impact crisis response and crisis management. First and foremost, the impact of constitutions, political regimes, and political institutions on crisis responsiveness is identifiable, in both small n and large N analyses, despite the many idiosyncrasies of individual country cases. Second, institutional history matters—provisions put in place either recently, following a previous crisis, or long in the past and almost forgotten through nonuse, come into play and either impede or empower decision makers, depending on how congruent they are with the de facto decision-making structures. Third,

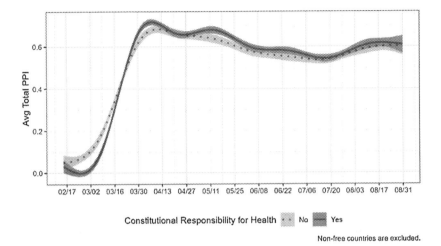

Fig. 10.10 Daily (average total) PPI in countries with and without a constitutionally specified right to health, February–August 2020. (Sources: Shvetsova et al. (2022), Freedom House (2020); author coding of constitutional responsibility for health.)

the economy imposes constraints on managing crises; not just the percapita income but the structure of the economy, the condition of the labor force, and the accumulated social capital are all prerequisites for mounting a more effective response. Fourth, political concerns of the day can make a huge difference: crisis response might be delayed because of immediate political expediency, or it might be hijacked and repurposed to solidify the position of political incumbents. Entering a crisis with a country's political "house" not "in order" is dangerous. Fifth, who does what in government—or the allocation of responsibilities—has shown itself to be a living, breathing process. It often underdoes rapid adjustments without recourse to formal institutional reforms or any open conflict over policy jurisdictions. Finally, the sixth and perhaps most important takeaway that all of this volume's contributors stress is that the mechanism through which all these influences affect the way governments respond to crises is by shaping the incentives of the key decision makers to act and take risks associated with leadership during periods of hardship. The resolve of politicians to protect public health cannot be taken for granted, and their strategies should be scrutinized at least as much through a political lens as from the standpoint of public health benefits.

REFERENCES

Adeel, A.B., Zhirnov, A. (2023). COVID-19 response in India, Pakistan, and Bangladesh: Shared history, different processes. In O. Shvetsova (Ed.), *Political institutions and governments' behavior in pandemic mitigation: Year 2020 around the world* (pp. ...). Springer Nature.

Bayar, M.C., Seyis, D. (2023). Populist responses to COVID-19: The cases of Turkey and Israel as examples of pro-science populism and the cases of the United States and Brazil as examples of science-skeptic populism. In O. Shvetsova (Ed.), *Political institutions and governments' behavior in pandemic mitigation: Year 2020 around the world* (pp. ...). Springer Nature.

Bayrali, O.G. (2023). Center-regional political risk sharing in COVID-19 public health crisis: Nigeria and South Africa. In O. Shvetsova (Ed.), *Political institutions and governments' behavior in pandemic mitigation: Year 2020 around the world* (pp. ...). Springer Nature.

Catalano, M., Chan, A. (2023). Common law systems and COVID-19 policy response: protective public health policy in the United States, Canada, New Zealand, and Australia. In O. Shvetsova (Ed.), *Political institutions and governments' behavior in pandemic mitigation: Year 2020 around the world* (pp. ...). Springer Nature.

Chu, H. (2023). The Visegrad populist leaders' responses to the pandemic in 2020. In O. Shvetsova (Ed.), *Political institutions and governments' behavior in pandemic mitigation: Year 2020 around the world* (pp. ...). Springer Nature.

Freedom House (2020). Freedom in the World. https://freedomhouse.org/sites/default/files/2020-02/2020_Country_and_Territory_Ratings_and_Statuses_FIW1973-2020.xlsx.

Gollier, C., 2001. Should we beware of the precautionary principle?. *Economic Policy, 16*(33), pp. 302–327.

Heller, W.B., Muftuoglu, E., Rosenberg, D. (2023). The institutional underpinnings of policy-making in the face of the COVID-19 pandemic in Europe. In O. Shvetsova (Ed.), *Political institutions and governments' behavior in pandemic mitigation: Year 2020 around the world* (pp. ...). Springer Nature.

Hooghe, L., Marks, G., Schakel A.H., Chapman Osterkatz, S., Niedzwiecki, S., Shair-Rosenfield, S. (2016). *Measuring Regional Authority*. Oxford University Press.

Mainwaring, S., Scully, T. (Eds.) (1995). *Building democratic institutions: Party systems in Latin America*. Stanford University Press.

Naushirvanov, T., Rosenberg, D., Sawyer, P., Seyis, D. (2022). How populists fuel polarization and fail their response to COVID-19: An empirical analysis. *Frontiers in Political Science, 4*.

Shair-Rosenfield, S., Schakel A.H.,, Niedzwiecki, S., Marks, G., Hooghe, L Chapman Osterkatz, S. (2020). Language difference and regional authority. Regional and Federal Studies, 31(1), 73–97.

Shvetsova, O. et al. (2022). "Protective Policy Index (PPI) global dataset of origins and stringency of COVID 19 mitigation policies." Scientific Data 9, 319.

The World Bank, World Development Indicators (2020). GNI per capita, PPP (constant 2017 international $). http://data.worldbank.org/indicator/NY.GNP.PCAP.PP.KD.

VanDusky-Allen, J. (2023). An Analysis of Government Responses to COVID-19 in Latin America's Three Federations. In O. Shvetsova (Ed.), *Political institutions and governments' behavior in pandemic mitigation: Year 2020 around the world* (pp. ...). Springer Nature.

Zhao, T. (2023). Pick your poison: Political expediencies, economic necessities, and COVID-19 response in Malaysia and Indonesia. In O. Shvetsova (Ed.), *Political institutions and governments' behavior in pandemic mitigation: Year 2020 around the world* (pp. ...). Springer Nature.

World Health Organization (2020a). Global Health Expenditure Database. https://apps.who.int/nha/database/Select/Indicators/en.

World Health Organization (2020b). World health statistics 2020: Monitoring health for the SDGs, sustainable development goals. https://www.who.int/publications/i/item/9789240005105.

APPENDIX A: PROTECTIVE POLICY INDEX (PPI) POLICY CATEGORIES AND ASSIGNED WEIGHTS (TABLES A.1 AND A.2)

Table A.1 Policy categories and their weights in PPI construction, method 1

Category	Variable	Weight in PPI
1. International and domestic air border closures	borders.air_bord	0.075
2. International and domestic land border closures	borders.land_bord	0.075
3. International and domestic sea border closures	borders.sea_bord	0.075
4. Limits on size of social gatherings	soc_and_schls. soc_gath	0.1
5. Closing of schools	soc_and_schls. schools	0.1
6. State of emergency	emerg.all	0.075
7. Closure of entertainment venues/stadiums	places.venues	0.025
8. Closure of restaurants	places.restrts	0.05
9. Closure of nonessential businesses	places.ne_busn	0.05
10. Closure of government offices	places.gov_offs	0.05
11. Work-from-home requirement for businesses/ organizations	places.wfh	0.025
12. Personal mobility restrictions	ind_locat.ind_mob	0.125
13. Self-isolation and/or quarantine requirements	ind_locat.med_stay	0.075
14. Public transportation closures	ind_locat.publ_tr	0.05
15. Mandatory wearing of PPE/masks	masks.all	0.05

© The Author(s), under exclusive license to Springer Nature Switzerland AG 2023
O. Shvetsova (ed.), *Government Responses to the COVID-19 Pandemic*, https://doi.org/10.1007/978-3-031-30844-4

244 APPENDIX A: PROTECTIVE POLICY INDEX (PPI) POLICY CATEGORIES...

Table A.2 Policy categories and their weights in Protective Policy Index construction, method 2

Category	Variable	Weight in PPI
1. International and domestic border closures	borders.all	0.110
2. Limits on size of social gatherings	soc_and_schls.soc_gath	0.110
3. Closing of schools	soc_and_schls.schools	0.110
4. State of emergency	emerg.all	0.041
5. Closure of entertainment venues/stadiums	places.venues	0.027
6. Closure of restaurants	places.restrts	0.055
7. Closure of nonessential businesses	places.ne_busn	0.055
8. Closure of government offices	places.gov_offs	0.055
9. Personal mobility restrictions	ind_locat.ind_mob	0.137
10. Self-isolation and/or quarantine requirements	ind_locat.med_stay	0.027
11. Quarantine	ind_locat.med_quar	0.055
12. Work-from-home requirement for businesses/organizations	places.wfh	0.027
13. Public transportation closures	ind_locat.pub_transp	0.055
14. Mandatory wearing of PPE/masks	med_mandate.masks	0.082
15. Personal distancing rules 1.5–2 m	med_mandate.dist_mand	0.055

Appendix B: Power Sharing and Stringency of Nonmedical Interventions (NMIs) (Figs. B.1, B.2, B.3, and B.4)

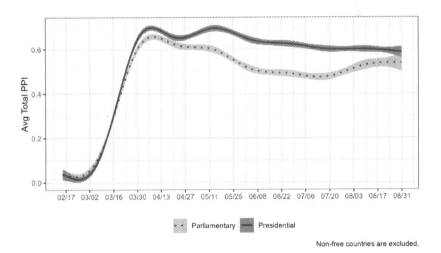

Fig. B.1 Daily (average total) Protective Policy Index in parliamentary (dotted) and presidential democracies, February–August 2020. (Source: Shvetsova et al. 2022)

© The Author(s), under exclusive license to Springer Nature Switzerland AG 2023
O. Shvetsova (ed.), *Government Responses to the COVID-19 Pandemic*, https://doi.org/10.1007/978-3-031-30844-4

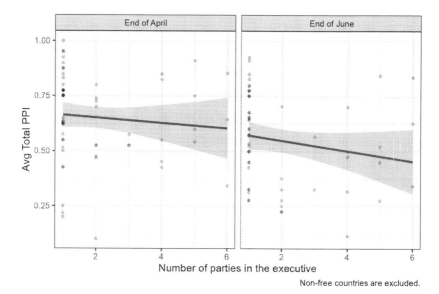

Fig. B.2 NMI stringency and power sharing in national executive. (Sources: Shvetsova et al. 2022; Döring, Huber, and Manow 2022)

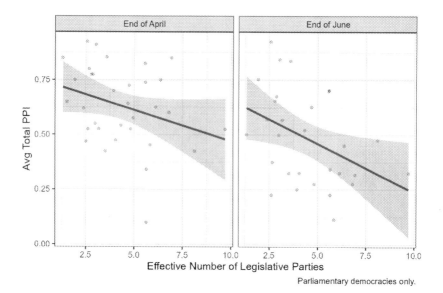

Fig. B.3 NMI stringency and multiparty systems in national legislatures, parliamentary democracies only. (Sources: Shvetsova et al. 2022; Döring et al. 2022)

APPENDIX B: POWER SHARING AND STRINGENCY OF NONMEDICAL... 247

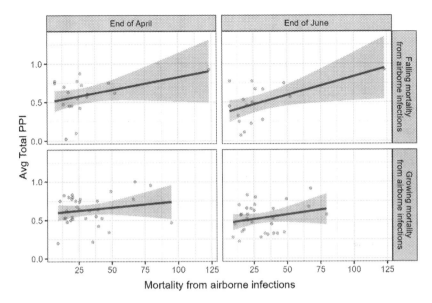

Fig. B.4 Correspondence between annual mortality from airborne infections (per 100,000) and NMI stringency, in countries with rising and declining mortality rates, in April and June 2020. (Sources: Shvetsova et al. 2022; WHO Mortality Database 2022)

INDEX[1]

A
Afghanistan, 91
Airports, 91
Andhra Pradesh, 89, 90
Argentina, 50–58, 63–66
Army, 84, 96, 97
Arunachal Pradesh, 89, 90, 93
Assam, 90, 93
Australia, 150, 198–205, 199n1, 203n5, 207–209, 212, 213n8, 214, 216–218
Awami League, 80
Azad Kashmir, 91, 93, 95

B
Babis, Andrej, 179
Baluchistan, 91, 93
Ban, 89, 90, 93
Bangladesh, 76–82, 84–87, 89, 92–96, 98–100, 102, 103

Department of Disaster Management, 85
Disaster Management Act 2012, 84
Disaster Management Advisory Committee, 84
Institute of Epidemiology, Disease Control and Research, 92
National Disaster Management Council (NDMC), 84
National Disaster Management Plan, 85
National Disaster Management Policy, 85
National Disaster Response Coordination Group, 85
Belgium, 18, 18n2
Bharatiya Janata Party (BJP), 80
Bhutan, 89
Bihar, 90, 93, 94
Biological and Public Health Emergencies, 83, 89

---

[1] Note: Page numbers followed by 'n' refer to notes.

© The Author(s), under exclusive license to Springer Nature Switzerland AG 2023
O. Shvetsova (ed.), *Government Responses to the COVID-19 Pandemic*, https://doi.org/10.1007/978-3-031-30844-4

249

250 INDEX

Blame avoidance, 160
Blame shifting, 24, 38
Bolsonaro, Jair, 57, 59, 61, 148, 149,
   152–155, 153n5, 157, 161, 162,
   167, 181
Bombay, 82, 100
Bombay Municipal Charter, 1888, 100
Border, 89, 91, 92
Brazil, 50–55, 57–64, 68, 148, 151,
   152, 154–157, 158n9, 159,
   161–167, 181, 182
The British Raj, 76, 77, 99–102
Bureaucracy, 198
Bureaucratic, *see* Bureaucracy

C
Cabinet, 18–20, 22, 23n4, 26, 27, 30,
   31, 34–38, 80
Calvary Chapel Dayton Valley v.
   Sisolak, 214, 215
Canada, 101, 118, 150, 198–208,
   199n1, 201n2, 212, 213n8,
   214–216, 218
Central Europe, 177
Chhattisgarh, 90
China, 89, 91
Cinemas, 90
Claiming credit, 19
Classification of interventions, 78
Coalition dynamics, 28
Common Law
   court, 95, 119n3, 199n1, 200–203,
      202n4, 203n5, 206–209, 211,
      213–217, 213n8, 219
   system, 99
Common pool problem, 22
Common-pool resources, 18
Community Mobility, 86
Containment, 76, 78, 89–92,
   94–97, 103

Containment zones, 90, 95, 96
The Constitution of India, 81
The Constitution of Pakistan, 81, 102
Court
   of Appeals, 200, 201, 213n8
   judiciary, 198
   justices, 201–203, 205,
      207–209, 219
   of last resort, 198–201, 203, 205,
      207–210, 212, 213, 213n8,
      215, 216, 218
   upheld, 95, 214–218
   writ of certiorari, 201
COVID-19, 6, 75–79, 85–104
Crisis management, 29, 113, 185,
   189, 191, 193
Critical juncture, 77, 98, 104
Czech Republic, 7, 177, 179, 188n8

D
Decentralization, 4, 138, 225–231
Delhi, 90, 93
Democratic accountability, 185
Denmark, 18, 18n2, 19, 24, 25, 27,
   28, 30, 34–35, 38–40
Department of Disaster
   Management, 86
Discussion and Concluding
   Remarks, 120–121

E
East India Company, 99
Economics, 19
The 18th Amendment, 81, 82, 102
Electoral costs, 179, 188, 190–193
Emergency, 82–85, 89, 91, 92, 100,
   101, 103
Epidemic Diseases Act, 1897, 77, 82,
   90, 93, 100, 102

INDEX   251

Europe, 18, 27, 29, 30, 32, 36, 38, 39, 101, 158
European Union, 18, 19, 114
Executive, 50, 80, 121, 162, 198, 199, 201, 204, 207, 209, 212, 214, 217, 218

F
February, 85, 86, 89–92
Federal, 76, 80–83, 90–92, 94–97, 99, 101–104
Federalism/federations, 29, 50, 56–58, 63, 69, 70, 75, 80, 96, 104, 120, 167
Finland, 18, 18n1, 18n2, 19, 24, 25, 27, 28, 30, 34–40
Free-riding, 75
Frente de Todos, 55

G
Gathering, 90, 92
Gerner v. Victoria, 216, 217
Gilgit-Baltistan, 91, 93, 95
Global Party Survey, 179n4
Goa, 89, 90, 93
Góes, Waldez, 60
Google Community Mobility reports, 86
Government of India Act 1935, 99
Governments multiparty, 19–24, 26, 27, 37, 50
Gujarat, 90, 93

H
Haryana, 90, 93
Hasina Wazed, Sheikh, 80
Healthcare system, 77, 80, 81, 102
Himachal Pradesh, 89, 90, 93

Historical institutionalism, 77, 98
H1N1, 68
Horizontal accountability, 185
Hungary, 7, 177, 177n1, 179, 180n5, 187, 188n8, 190

I
Ideology, 77, 151, 151n3, 198, 203, 205, 207–209, 219
India, 76–87, 89–94, 96–103
Disaster Management Act, 2005, 83, 84
Ministry of Home Affairs, 92
National Disaster Management Authority (NDMA), 83, 89, 92
National Disaster Management Plan, 2019, 83
National Disaster Response Force (NDRF), 83
National Executive Committee (NEC), 83
National Policy on Disaster Management, 2009, 83
Indian National Congress (INC), 80
Indonesia, 7, 127–143, 229
The Infectious Diseases (Prevention, Control and Elimination) Act, 2018, 82
Institutional legacies, 178, 192
Introduction, 107–110
Iran, 89, 91
Italy, 18, 18n1, 19, 24, 25, 27, 29–32, 31n6, 34, 35, 37, 39, 40, 89

J
Janata curfew, 92
January, 85, 86, 89–92
Jharkhand, 90, 94
Johnson, Boris, 181

252 INDEX

Judiciary, 34, 104, 198, 200–204, 205n6, 207, 211, 213n8, 215, 219
Juntos por el Cambio, 55
Jurisdiction/jurisdictions, 19–23, 23n4, 37, 38, 81, 85, 113, 121, 200–203, 213n8, 215, 216

K
Karnataka, 90
Kerala, 89, 90
Khan, Imran, 80, 94
Khyber Pakhtunkhwa, 91, 95

L
Legislative, 20, 27, 35, 59, 120, 198, 201, 204, 217
Lockdown, 86, 92–97

M
Madhya Pradesh, 90, 93
Maharashtra, 90
Majority coalition, 19, 20, 31, 35
Malaysia, 7, 127–143, 229, 234
Malls, 90, 93
March, 76, 85, 86, 89–94, 103
Matovic, Igor, 179
The Ministry of National Health Services, Regulation and Coordination, 81–82
Morawiecki, Mateusz, 179
May, 76, 87, 94–97
Mexico, 50–55, 57, 62–69, 63n1, 151, 151n3
Military, 76, 85, 92, 94, 97, 103, 104
Ministers, 21, 84, 92
Ministry of Health and Family Welfare, 81
Mizoram, 90, 93

Modi, Narendra, 80
MORENA, 65, 66
Myanmar, 89, 92

N
Nagaland, 90
National, 75, 80–84, 86, 89, 92, 94–97, 99, 103
National Democratic Alliance, 80
National Disaster Management Plan, 83, 86, 89
National Institute of Health, 91, 92
Nepal, 89
Netherlands, the, 18
New Zealand, 198–205, 199n1, 202n3, 207, 208, 212, 213n8, 214, 216, 218
Nigeria, 108–114, 120, 121
The 1958 Epidemic Diseases Act for West Pakistan, 82
Non-medical interventions, 78, 86, 97, 101
mitigation policies, 57, 58, 68, 70
protective policies, 148–150, 153n5, 155, 156, 159–162, 167, 168, 212, 213n8, 217
variation, 97, 223

O
Odisha, 90, 93
Orban, Viktor, 179

P
Pakistan, 76–82, 84–87, 89–93, 95–103
District Disaster Management Authorities (DDMA), 84
Field Epidemiology and Disease Surveillance Division, 91

INDEX 253

National Action Plan, 92
National Command and Operation Center (NCOC), 94, 97
National Coordination Committee, 94, 95
National Disaster Management Act, 2010, 84
National Disaster Management Authority (NDMA), 84
National Disaster Management Ordinance, 2006, 84
National Disaster Response Force (NDRF), 83
National Executive Commission (NEC), 84
National Institute of Health, 90
Provincial Disaster Management Authorities (PDMA), 84
Supreme Court, 95
Pakistan Muslim League (Nawaz), 80
Pakistan Peoples Party (PPP), 80
Pakistan Tehreek-e-Insaf (PTI), 80
Parliamentarism, 4
Parliamentary, 19, 24, 26–28, 30, 32, 35, 38, 39, 41, 80, 115, 119, 157
Parties
  number of parties, 18–20, 22, 26, 30, 41
Partisanship, 50, 62, 68, 205
Party system/party systems, 18, 50, 55, 58, 59, 62, 65, 70, 110, 111, 115, 121, 200, 203, 204, 207
Path dependence, 77, 98, 98n2
Plague, 82, 100, 101
Poland, 7, 177, 177n1, 179, 180n5, 186, 187, 188n8, 190
Political conflict, 76
Population density, 18, 26, 29, 167
Populism, 148–151, 166, 167, 179, 179n4, 183
Populist, 150–155, 167, 179n4, 183, 190
Precedent, 198–202, 209, 210, 212, 214, 215

Pre-emptive, 89
Prime Minister, 83, 84, 89, 92, 94, 95
Protective Policy Index (PPI), 49–52, 60, 63n1, 66, 67, 86, 89n1, 108, 109, 156, 159, 162–166
  components, 9, 162
Public health, 6, 76–79, 81–83, 88, 92, 96–98, 100–104
Public transport, 93
Punjab, 90, 91, 93, 95

Q
Quarantine, 82, 89–92, 95

R
Rajasthan, 90, 93
The responsibility for healthcare, 81
Restrictions, 78, 87, 89, 90, 93–96, 101, 104
Roman Catholic Diocese of Brooklyn v. Cuomo, 214, 215

S
Saudi Arabia, 91
Schools, 90, 91, 96
Screening, 92
Section 144, 90, 91
Self-isolation, 89, 93
Semashko health care system, 178, 178n2, 188
Shifting blame, *see* Blame avoidance
Sindh, 82, 91, 93, 95, 97
Sindh Epidemic Diseases Act, 2014, 82
Slovakia, 18
Smart lockdown, 95
Social distancing, 93, 94
Social gatherings, 90, 91
South Africa, 108–110, 112, 115–121
South Bay United Pentecostal Church v. Newsom, 214

254 INDEX

South Korea, 89
Spain, 18, 18n1, 18n2, 19, 24, 25, 27, 29–30, 32–35, 37, 39, 40
State, 80, 82–84, 89, 90, 93–96, 99, 103
Stringency, 27, 28, 49–51, 59, 60, 62, 63, 63n1, 67–69, 85, 86, 101, 108, 164, 165
Subnational, 76, 80–82, 86, 90, 93, 96, 97, 102–104
Supreme Court, 76, 97

T
Theaters, 90
Thermal screening, 91
Timing, 29
Tragedy of the commons, 22
Travel, 89, 92, 94
Trump, Donald, 148, 149, 152–155, 153n4, 153n5, 161, 162, 166, 167, 181, 206

U
Union Ministry of Health and Family Welfare, 81, 90
Unitary, 80, 99

United Kingdom, the, 178n3, 181
United States, 152, 155, 158n9, 161–166, 181, 198, 199n1, 200–207, 213–215, 213n8
Unlock 1.0, 95
Unlock 2.0, 95
Unlock 3.0, 95
Uttarakhand, 89
Uttar Pradesh, 90

V
Vaccination, 78, 89, 101
Vaccines, 78, 89
Visegrad, 177, 177n1, 178, 186, 189, 192

W
West Bengal, 90
WHO, *see* World Health Organization
Workforce, 39, 64, 178n2, 180, 192
World Health Organization (WHO), 81, 82, 95, 102, 104

Z
Zema, Romeu, 60

Printed in the United States
by Baker & Taylor Publisher Services